YOU KNOW WHAT IT'S LIKE

By Barbara Cunningham

Barbara Cunningham

Published by
Chipmunkapublishing
PO Box 6872
Brentwood
Essex CM13 1ZT
United Kingdom

http://www.chipmunkapublishing.com

YOU DON'T KNOW WHAT IT'S LIKE

The Author.. My Mum

My Mum, Barbara Cunningham, is a fabulous if at times slightly eccentric mother of a beautiful, witty intelligent daughter and a ginger son. Educated at Keele University, she holds a dual honours Bachelor of Science degree in Psychology and Criminology, as well as various slightly less orthodox qualifications including Culinary Arson Studies.

With a career history that borders on chameleonic, her lines of work have included journalism, insurance broking, running a pub, being the life and soul of the staff party at the Keele University Nuffield Library (a surprisingly tall order) and most recently putting the youth of our nation on the straight and narrow as part of the Essex Youth Offending Team.

A keen badminton and netball player, she even had a stint playing for and managing a netball team who, while not perhaps being the most feared opponents in the land, were nonetheless the envy of the Chelmsford league for being such a thoroughly nice bunch of girls!

Whilst this is her first literary publication, she has high hopes of writing a host of Pulitzer Prize winners in the future. Possible titles include 'The Carbon Cookbook' and '100 Ways to Shut Your Daughter Up: A Practical Guide to Domestic Serenity'.

I might never have told her, but now she can see it in print, that I am one of her biggest fans. I admire her for her endurance, for her courage and for her strength. I admire her for the care and guidance she gave to her offspring when she would have desperately needed someone to guide and care for her, and I admire her for her selflessness and durability. But most of all I admire her for never giving up and for giving so much love to those she loved even though she was so often deprived of it herself.

Mum, you are really cool and I love you ... loads.

Victoria

Acknowledgements

My children, Daniel and Victoria, for surviving my parenting and cooking.

My beautiful sisters, Colleen and Susan, for their love and continued support.

Jonathan Ashby, who nagged and bullied me into writing this book but also encouraged and gave me the confidence to complete it.

Paula, for the love, laughter, tears and brandy, you were always there for me.

My netball friends for the food, the clothing, the babysitting and the hangovers!

My netball friends husbands, past and present, for doing as they were told.

Katie Lachter, for believing in me even when I didn't believe in myself.

Keele University for not turning me away.

Tesco for buy one get one free.

Matalan for the inexpensive, quality clothing.

Jim, Tony, Colin and Derek for helping me ease back into the terrifying world of dating, well... maybe not Derek!

Jason Pegler for saying yes to my book

Barbara Cunningham

YOU DON'T KNOW WHAT IT'S LIKE

CHAPTERS

Barbara Cunningham

YOU DON'T KNOW WHAT IT'S LIKE

I sat on her comfortable leather sofa, trying not to caress it lovingly with my finger tips and asked her politely to please turn off her television. I say 'television' but this thing was HUGE – COLOSSAL – MASSIVE – and any other descriptive word you could think of. My complete family could have moved into it and not bumped into each other for days. OK, I'm exaggerating, but it was quite the largest television I had ever seen in my life!

"You don't know what it's like," she sobbed into her glass of whatever. "I've got three boys, I live on bloody Income Support – bet you don't even know what that is – I only get £300 a month from me ex but at least that's in cash and me nerves are a wreck 'case benefits find out about it and me bar work!!"

On and on she droned, only pausing to take another drag on her cigarette or to shout at Tom, Dick or Harry to shut the f*** up … I'm busy … play on your computers!

I walked away from the house with the sound of her screaming at her unruly children ringing in my ears. How many more times was I going to be told 'you don't know what it's like?' How many more times would I be forced to bite my tongue for the sake of the policies and protocols demanded by my bosses at the Youth Offending Service?

'I *do* know what it's like!' I wanted to shout.

The difference?   I wasn't tame, I wasn't complacent, I was a feisty, gobby, mother cat who fought for her rights and the rights of her children. I did everything I could to crawl out of the poverty trap. I'd been to hell and back, looked poverty and prejudice in the face and stuck my fingers up at both of them.

Want to know how I did it? Well read my story!

YOU DON'T KNOW WHAT IT'S LIKE

THE BEGINNING

For four hours he had been beating me – throwing me around the kitchen as if I weighed nothing – dragging me upstairs to the bedroom, shouting, slapping, punching and throwing! I was too exhausted to feel pain anymore, too afraid for my children to worry about my own safety. When would it stop … please God make him stop!!

"I can't even shout at you anymore," roared Bob, my furious, drunken husband, but the roar trailed off into a pathetic shriek as he clutched his strained throat.

There was a tiny tap-tap-tap at the bedroom door. Bob threw it open, and there, white faced, huge scared eyes, stood our tiny, 5 year old son, David, in his shaking hands he clutched two, heavy pint glasses brimming over with milk. He looked from his father's furious face to mine, looked with unconcealed horror at my cut lip, swollen bleeding nose, black eyes, rapidly swelling cheeks …

"Daddy, you're not hurting mummy are you?" he asked in a tiny incredulous, terrified voice.

With that Bob's temper seemed to dissipate, his eyes lost that manic look. Staggering, he took the milk from our son's weakening grip and in a gentle voice he said, "Of course not boy, now go look after your sister," as he slowly closed the door on David's horrified and disbelieving face.

I shrank back and as he turned to me and reached out his hand, I stumbled and fell onto the bed. Did he think that was an invitation? He threw himself next to me tearing at my already ripped nightdress, "That's what I want, make love to me, show me you love me," he gasped, as I struggled not to turn my head away from his rancid hot breath.

'I *can* do this – I *must* do this,' I thought, and I did. For what seemed an eternity, I crawled out of my body and watched from a distance, as my other self made love to this man and as he climaxed and drew me to him with a look of love on his face, I said to him, in a silent voice, "You lose – you lose me, your children, your home and your business". And just for the most fleeting of moments, I felt a terrible sorrow for the man I had once loved.

ON THE RUN

Where could I go, what was I going to do? I was driving away from my best friend's flat. She had been half awake. It was still only 6 o'clock in the morning. Kate had looked with horror at my swollen, bruised and bleeding face. The children had clung to her, their eyes full of fright.

"You must stay here," she pleaded.

"I can't, I can't, he will look for me here first … he will expect me to come here. I need to leave NOW … I just couldn't leave without telling you first… he will contact you … looking for me … I know he will. I must go!!"

Kate had thrown biscuits and sweets and crisps into a plastic bag and all the money she could find … she was crying, softly. How many others would be hurt by my drunken husband's violence? I hated this, I HATED IT!!

We hugged her and I promised to contact her as soon as I had found somewhere to stay and then we fled Braintree, the town I had lived in for over 20 years.

The children slept, at last, in the back of the car. My 2 ½ year old daughter, Louise, was showing signs of fever, her little cheeks were flushed, her breathing laboured. In her sleep she clung to her brother. Occasionally, David whimpered. I felt my heart would break, would he forget what he had seen and heard, or would he carry this with him for the rest of his life?

I needed to think, I had to go somewhere where I could think! I drove to Mersea Island, a place I had always loved, a tiny unspoiled island off the Essex coast, near Colchester.

The children played in the sand whilst I sat and allowed myself to silently weep. I had washed the blood from my face with the salty water and now it was throbbing painfully. I called the children to me and they ate some of the food Kate had given us, whilst I counted the money. My money and Kate's came to £40, where would we stay with so little? Louise stroked my face with amazing gentleness, "Poor mummy, I'll kiss it all better." It was strange that she hadn't asked what had happened to me. Her tiny body felt so hot, I needed somewhere to stay and soon, she was definitely sickening for something. David hugged me, his eyes showed such sadness I could hardly bare it. He loved his father so much, had already in his few years, forgiven him for breaking many promises. Would he forgive him this also?

Louise slept again as we drove into Colchester. I tried several places before a couple, John and Mary Richards, running a tiny hotel on North Hill, took pity on us and gave us a room for the night for only £5. After hearing my story, John hid my car at the back of the hotel and then moved a cot into the room for Louise. Mary chatted to David whilst she busied herself in the cosy kitchen, making the children something to eat and giving me the opportunity to phone Kate. My dear friend had been busy. She had contacted our friends and together they had booked us a caravan to stay in on Mersea Island. We could go there the next morning.

I allowed myself to hope that things would be alright. Kate hadn't heard from Bob – I wasn't that surprised – he had been so drunk he would probably still be asleep, blissfully unaware of the drama he had created.

It was now midday and I was dreadfully tired, I could barely keep my eyes open.

"Go sleep," said Mary, "I'll feed the children and watch them for you, your little girl will probably need to sleep too."

Reluctantly but desperate for sleep, I left the children with Mary and John and went to our room. My eyes filled with tears when I found they had put toys in the room for the children, there was a box of Lego, a little doll, paper and crayons, children's books.

Also, carefully laid out on a clean cloth, was antiseptic and cotton wool for me to take care of my damaged face. There was shampoo, soap, toothpaste and toothbrushes – in my panic to leave Braintree I hadn't packed anything, all we had were the clothes we were wearing. I also noticed a comb and hair brush and I finally collapsed on the bed sobbing, when under the hairbrush, I saw a £5 note.

MAKING PLANS

That night, whilst the children slept, I started to make plans. I felt mentally and physically stronger having had a couple of hours fitful sleep and Louis's fever seemed to have broken. That had been a real concern to me, although it hadn't really appeared to have bothered her at all.

I knew, at this stage, I needed help. I couldn't do this on my own but who or what could I turn too?

Maybe illogically, I phoned the Samaritans. Looking back, I think I felt my story was so shocking, so horrible, only the Samaritans would be able to listen and advise me.

I had made a really good choice. Adam listened silently as my story spilled out.

"I'm not suicidal," I promised him, "I just need advice, need help, someone to talk to, someone to listen to me."

Adam asked about the children, carefully checking on their safety and health.

Then he calmly talked to me ... what were my injuries? Was anything broken? Did I need money? Was I strong enough to carry on tonight – make some more calls? Oh yes, I was strong enough now and resolute!!

Adam gave me the telephone numbers of several 'Battered Wives Homes' – now thankfully known as 'Women's Refuges' – *battered wives* sounds like something you buy from the chippie, no dignity in that!! He also suggested I call into their office in Colchester the next morning, if I still needed support.

YOU DON'T KNOW WHAT IT'S LIKE

We talked for a little longer, I loved his calm gentle voice but I knew there could be other calls more urgent than mine, so I thanked him for his kindness and with tears hot in my eyes, said goodbye. God was I going to cry every time someone was kind to me?

I phoned several refuges. Shockingly, none in Essex had any spare rooms! However, a kind lady at the Colchester Refuge gave me the telephone number of a local solicitor, well known for her support of women 'in my position' – 'beaten black and blue,' I thought, cynically.

The manager of the Greys refuge said she may have an available room the next day but added, "Mrs Cunningham, you sound very strong, have a good night's sleep, maybe tomorrow you will find you don't need us!"

As I crawled off to bed I wondered what she had meant by that. I stared into the bedroom mirror – Quasimodo stared back and then I *knew* what she'd meant! No battered wives home for me, onward and upward ... get the bastard out of the house ... get the children home ... get a divorce!! Anger was now edging its way into my psyche!!

The next morning Mary made the three of us delicious breakfasts then, somewhat embarrassed, she gave me two bags of clothing for the children. She had been up very early and had begged, stolen and borrowed clothes from her friends and family. For me, she had some of her own clothing. As she was 5' 6" and about 16 stone and I was 5' 1" and around 9 stone, this at last gave us all something to laugh about! I paraded around the kitchen in her ill fitting outfits, finally settling on a pair of jeans rolled up at the ankles, the waist drawn in tightly by a wide, heavily studded leather belt in which John had hastily made extra holes, and one of John's smallest shirts tucked in at the waste.

"Mummy," said Louise, "You look like a *BionicBabs*!" I could only assume my badly bruised, swollen face and the large studded belt had made her think this. Whatever her reason, this nickname later became a fairly large part of my life!!

We left the security of the hotel having said an emotional goodbye to John and Mary. I really hoped one day I would be able to tell them how much they had helped us with their total selfless kindness.

I had made further plans and my first trip was to the Samaritan's office in Elm Lane, Colchester. The staff there volunteered to look after the children to allow me the opportunity to visit the recommended local solicitor.

Sitting in a huge, bright and airy office, the walls decorated with her framed certificates and diplomas, Jasmine McCarthy looked as if she had only recently left school, however, she proved to be very wise and an expert at her profession. She listened in silence to my story, a story I was sure she had heard many times before. She made rapid neat notes in a numbered notebook, the cover headed, 'Barbara Cunningham (40) DV'!

The nightmare story reduced me to tears yet again, 'would they never dry up?' I thought to myself. She first handed me a tissue then finally pushed the whole box in my direction.

"Put them in your bag," she said, "If you do as I tell you, this is going to be a difficult and emotional day but I promise you, I will have you home within a week, and an injunction against your husband within 48 hours"!!

Jasmine pushed her phone and a piece of paper with the name and telephone number of a female Doctor on Mersea Island, toward me. As she left her office she said to me, "Make an appointment, preferably for today!!"

The full horror of what I had to do suddenly hit me. She wanted photographic proof of my injuries. Swallowing what was left of my pride I dialled the number and made an appointment for 3pm that same afternoon.

MERSEA ISLAND AND MY FRIENDS

The drive to Mersea had been in silence, the children seemingly aware that mummy didn't want to talk.

As we drove onto the island I was aware that for the first time ever, my spirits were not lifted by its unspoiled serenity and beauty. The children and I had visited Mersea often, it was the place we would come to when my husband was on one of his drinking binges and would disappear for days on end. Many, many times I had thought 'this time he may not be drinking, he may have had an accident and be lying injured in a ditch somewhere.' On those occasions, whatever the time of night, I would put the children, wrapped up warm and cosy in their baby seats in the back of my car and we would go play, 'Hunt the Daddy,' turning my ordeal into a game for them.

At that time, we were running a small business, selling charcoal to Indian restaurants. Bob was out all hours delivering the charcoal and collecting the money. My job was to get new business and keep the books, something I proved to be extremely adept at.

'Hunt the Daddy' involved driving to all his delivery points and then, hopefully, taking what I believed to be his route home. However, my journey more recently had been to drive past the homes of his friends throughout Romford and Ilford, the children peering through the often steamed up windows of my badly heated car, looking for daddy's big white

YOU DON'T KNOW WHAT IT'S LIKE

van. When it was spotted the children would scream with delight, "We win we win, there's daddy's van!"

I would resist banging on the door of the house, well aware of the violence Bob was capable of when drunk and cornered.

Instead we would drive home and the children would number, date and enter the details into a little book and I would promise to tell daddy when the figure reached 100, that they were the winners of a game he knew nothing about.

The small amount of money we were making was, more often than not, spent on his 'evenings out.' I was constantly short of money and it was my dear friend Kate who, uncritically, often brought food around and fed the children.

We knew instantly which caravan had been booked for us, for outside one overlooking the sea, were several parked cars. I ran a netball club in Braintree and Kate had arrived, mob handed, with several of our friends. They had a barbeque burning and were busy turning the caravan into what was to be our home for the next seven days.

The girls were shocked when they saw the mess my face was in, "Don't worry," I said, "I won, look – I have the belt to prove it!" Somewhat hysterical laughter followed – only Kate stood on the periphery as she held my two children, who loved her so much, to her, her eyes full of tears.

The girls had thought of everything. Amongst the goodies they had brought with them were two large bottles of wine, more food than I had seen in months, make-up, plasters, buckets and spades, even a box of tampons and 200 cigarettes.

Kate came with me to the doctors whilst the others played on the beach with the children. It was the most beautiful April day, but I failed miserably to pretend we were on holiday.

I would never ever forgive my husband the humiliation that followed. I had to strip naked, every inch of my body was examined and photographed, poked and prodded. I had to bend this way and that to prove difficulty of mobility caused by several bruised ribs and strained stomach muscles. There were dark finger bruises on my arms, thighs and shins where he had pinned me to the bed, bites on my neck, breasts and shoulders. Close up photographs were taken of my face, my nose, twice its size, was luckily not broken. The doctor laid down the camera and looked sadly at me. "You should see the other guy," I said, with a pathetic attempt at humour.
"Mrs Cunningham, I want you to keep copies of these pictures, just in case you are ever tempted to return to him."
"If I do," I replied, "you have my permission to shoot me!!"

When Kate and I returned to the caravan the children were asleep, cuddled up together, looking so tiny and vulnerable on the double bed, holding tightly onto their newly acquired soft toys.

YOU DON'T KNOW WHAT IT'S LIKE

The girls naturally wanted to know what had happened. I told them I'd been sleeping in the spare room for some weeks, biding my time and planning my escape from a miserable marriage. I'd awoken at 4 a.m. – was it only the previous morning – to the sounds of excited squeals from David and Louise. I had gone downstairs and found Bob staggering drunkenly around the kitchen. He'd looked at me through glazed, empty eyes and told me he was taking the children to Alton Towers for the day. It was at this point that I knew I was in for a beating, for I had to stop him driving away with our precious children. I'd calmly said ... "No you are not" ... and with that the attack had begun.

Several hours later, the girls drove away, promising to return as soon as they could. Only Kate stayed, typical of her, she had taken a week off work to be with the children and me.

Unable to sleep, we talked all night, and then took it in turns the next day to look after the children whilst the other slept. The following morning I drove back to Colchester to see Jasmine, carrying with me the horrid photographs.
She told me that Bob would have already received the injunction and been given 5 days, by a judge, to leave the family home.
My spirits lifted, I drove back to Mersea and joyfully told Kate the children and I would be home on Sunday.

Suddenly a tiny, scared voice said "Mummy!" and I turned to see David standing petrified in the doorway of the caravan, his little hand turning blue in the furious grip of his father's!

I bent down and put my arms out to my son, "Come here sweetie," I said, smiling gently at him, "Come to mummy, daddy won't hurt you." Bob relaxed his grip and David broke free, rushing up the steps of the caravan into my arms. I held him closely to me feeling his little heart pounding in his chest as if it would burst through.

"Daddy, are you going to stay with us and play in the sand"? Louise asked as she came into the room rubbing her sleepy eyes. I gently pushed David toward Kate and picking Louise up placed her into Kate's protective arms. "Take the children into the back of the van Kate". She began to argue but I shook my head, "Take them, I'll be fine."

"I wanna talk to my fuckin' kids," shouted Bob.

I spun wildly around – heaven knows what he saw in my eyes for he backed away from the steps of the caravan. I stood in the doorway, for once looking down on him. I didn't shout, I didn't even raise my voice. What came out was more like a hiss …

"You want … *you* want!! What you want is no longer a concern of this family, I couldn't give a *damn* what you want … but what *I* want is for you to get the fuck out of here before SOMEONE CALLS THE POLICE" – this last bit I shouted at the top of my voice. I hugged my ribs and almost screamed in pain, a tiny drop of blood dripped from my nose onto the back of my hand. This incensed me even more, reminding me of the fear and pain he had put me through only three days ago. I went down the steps of the caravan and slowly approached him. To my amazement he backed off again – not so brave when he wasn't full of booze.

"I will see you in court Bob, until then I don't want to see your face or hear your voice again, now GO!!"

In the distance could clearly be heard, the sound of police cars approaching the campsite.

Bob hesitated for just a moment "I found you here, I will find you again", he growled.

"No need to go searching," I replied, with as much humour in my voice as I could muster. "I'll be home," I smiled. "And there will be copies of the court injunction pasted on every wall and every fence of the house."

As he turned to go I said, "Oh and the children won the 'Hunt the Daddy' game 30 times."

"What the fuck's that?" he shouted.

"Oh you'll find out," I smiled, "you'll find out"!

With that I turned and carefully climbed back into the caravan, holding onto my throbbing ribs. I closed the door behind me and locked it, 'the worm has turned' I thought, 'the worm has most definitely turned!'

THAT'S WHAT FRIENDS ARE FOR

The children clung onto me as I unlocked the door. My hand was shaking. What the hell was wrong with me – this was our home! I pushed the door open, half expecting Bob to come rushing at me. Nothing, the house was silent … smelt … what *was* that dreadful smell?

Kate, standing next to me, said "Oh hell!"

Not letting them into the house I said, "Take the kids to the park Kate".

"C'mon kids, lets get some ice cream and see if any of your friends are down the park," she said, taking their hands and leading them out of the garden.

The children weren't bothered about the house. The park and friends and of course ice cream, were far more tempting. As they left the garden I bolted the gate behind them. The bolt was stiff and rusty, 'hmm' I thought, 'I've never used that before'. It was the first of many things I started to do that I had never done before.

The kitchen was a mess, broken glass and crockery all over the floor. I had a flashback of Bob picking me up and throwing me against a cupboard, the doors above thrown open by the force and the contents smashing to the floor.

The smell was now making me heave. Nearest the door was the waste bin, I didn't look inside, simply lifted it up and carried it to the back of the garden.

Back in the kitchen I ventured forward, my heart in my mouth … there was vomit mixed in with the broken glass. Stepping further in I noticed dried blood on the arch leading to the hall … 'my blood', I thought, fighting back the memory of him grabbing my hair and pushing me into the hall as I grabbed the side of the arch to stop myself falling.

More dried vomit in the hall, I glanced to my right, the dining room appeared undamaged, I wanted to throw open the French doors but fear of him suddenly appearing stopped me.

The next room on the right was the lounge. Shattered ornaments lay on the marble hearth – ornaments he had swept from the fire-surround in his rage, as I stood rigid with fear in the hall, holding onto the banister of the stairs for support – more dried blood bearing testament.

There were empty bottles scattered over the floor, cans on the coffee table, empty food cartons everywhere, more vomit, the constant sickening smell of urine.

Fear gripping me, I ventured upstairs but only got as far as our bedroom. On the bedside table were two pint glasses, one full of rancid milk, the other empty. The bed was a mess and again stunk of urine, the filthy sheets covered in my dried blood. Something else was there. I forced myself to look closer, my hand going to the back of my head, still, after seven days, incredibly tender. There, in the mess and the blood, was a perfect clump of my hair.

I almost fell as I rushed down the stairs and back outside, into the warm fresh air, sobbing, fighting back nausea, gasping for breath, perspiration pouring down my face … how was I ever going to feel safe here again, turn this house back into a family home?

My heart froze as a hand suddenly appeared over the top of the gate feeling for the bolt – but it was only Kate, shouting to be let in.

She sat with me on the overgrown grass, "You look like shit," she said.

"You're no oil painting yourself," I replied and we both fell about laughing and crying and holding onto each other like only true friends can.

She had left the children with Jayne, another friend, who had been at the park with her two children.

"She's going to feed and bathe them," said Kate. "We have about three hours to put things right."

"You pour in the petrol and throw in the lighted match and I'll call the fire brigade in about six hours," I said.

Again we collapsed into uncontrollable, hysterical laughter.

Kate left me in the garden whilst she went back into the house to do what she called a 'recce.'

She reappeared 10 minutes later with a scarf tied around her nose and mouth and wearing dark glasses.

"That bad?" I asked but smiled recognising the humour.

"Well," she said, "Bob has given a whole new meaning to 'having a bit of a piss up.' I've stripped your bed then I phoned some of our more strong stomached friends to give us a hand."

Sure enough, we could already hear cars pulling up outside and through the gate came nearly all the members of my own and other netball clubs with husbands and boyfriends in tow. I allowed the tears to flow once again as one by one my dear friends gently hugged me.

Wearing rubber gloves going up to the elbows, and several of them wearing 'wellies', armed with brushes and brooms, vacuum cleaners, carpet cleaners, antiseptic, scrubbing brushes etc, they set to work and in the background "That's What Friends Are For" played over and over again on the stereo.

Hours later, when I was alone, the children sound asleep in bed, the house sparkling and smelling like a hospital, panic started to overwhelm me. I had checked every door and window over and over again but it just wasn't enough. I searched for rope, string, belts, old washing line, skipping ropes, bootlaces, anything I could tie together. Then I wove an intricate web, attaching door to window, from the dining room to the hall, then back to the kitchen and from the kitchen to the lounge, pulling as tight as I could until, at last, I was sure no one could gain entrance from outside. Then I crawled onto the sofa and slept and there I slept, every night, for the next six months.

A DAY IN COURT

We were divorced within two months. His day in court was his last attempt at control. To my utter dismay he had decided to *fight* the divorce, arriving with a barrister and a string of 'mates' who would take to the stand in turn and swear what a wonderful husband and father he was. His pièce de résistance was the production of architectural plans for our house, dividing it into two flats. He stated he would live in the top flat and the children and I could take the ground floor flat. "That way," he declared, "I can continue to see my wife and children and carry on running the family business."

I was called back to the stand, the judge looked at me with some sympathy, "Mrs Cunningham, how do you feel about this, it would indeed keep the family together?"

I felt the blood drain from my face, 'my God,' I thought, 'he's actually considering this'!

As a young journalist, I had spent many years in court and had drawn on that experience. Seeing off his 'witnesses' – declaring that they were his drinking and gambling buddies with no knowledge of him as a father and a husband – I added, with as much dignity as I could muster, "But I do accept that they know him, in some ways better than his own children, as they have spent more time with him."

Now I looked the judge squarely in the eyes, "Sir," I said, strength and determination returning to my voice, "I would leave, I will not spend one more night under the same roof as this man, I would take my children and I would leave!"

As I walked on unsteady legs back to my seat, the judge asked my husband to stand up.

"Mr Cunningham, your wife has had enough, I am granting her the divorce, you will have to go to the Family Court and find other ways of seeing your children but this marriage is now over"!

I rushed from the court. I wanted to be with my children, I couldn't wait to start our new lives, free of fear, free of heartbreak and disappointment. We would be alright. I would make sure of that, we *would* be alright. Little did I know!

DARKNESS DESCENDS

I looked in dismay at the money in front of me £22 Family Allowance + £86 Income Support, that made £108 a week for the children and me to live on, to pay all the household bills except mortgage and council tax. This had to pay for food, clothing and shoes, 'bind their feet' I thought cynically. Then there was the car, there was the tax, insurance, petrol, oil, MOT, repairs. There were repairs to the house that needed paying for, the drains kept blocking up and sewage was flowing into the garden, not just our sewage. We were the end of the row and other householders were simply pushing their waste along the sewage pipes until it finally found an exit in our garden. The council refused to do the repairs to the antiquated drainage system, as this was not council property. Then there was a very worrying growth of moss along a crack in the damp course of the house. This went all the way around the outside wall of the kitchen. I was sure, somewhere underneath the kitchen floor, a pipe was slowly leaking.

Inside the house, damp was showing in Louise's bedroom. I had been forced to throw away pictures from her walls where the frames were rotting with mildew. And neither Louise nor David could see through their bedroom windows. The seal in the double-glazing was somewhere breaking down and between the two pains of glass, was thick condensation.

YOU DON'T KNOW WHAT IT'S LIKE

I had loved this barn of a house as soon as I had seen it four years earlier. We had been living in a first floor flat when David was born. It had been such a struggle to do anything, leaving him in the flat on his own whilst I carried the pram down the stairs, then dashing back for him, convinced that he had learned to walk the second he was out of my site. We didn't have a garden, so the hot weather meant going somewhere every day to escape the heat of the flat. It doesn't sound much but every mother will know it meant – the dreaded baby box being dragged along with spare nappies, cream, wipes, bibs, a change of clothing, food, drink, toys … the list was endless.

So this rambling, four bedroom, detached house with its small back and front gardens, within walking distance of Braintree town centre, was an absolute luxury. It was in desperate need of TLC when we bought it – many of the lathe and plaster walls and ceilings displaying frightening cracks – and there were polystyrene tiles on every ceiling. I wasn't concerned. Bob, a jack-of-all-trades, master of none, had promised to 'do the house up,' after all we had the rest of our lives in which to do it.

Of course it never happened. Bob would start a job, hit a problem and then disappear for days on end, leaving me to cope with the chaos he left in his wake.

On the day we moved into the house, with full packing cases everywhere, armed with a crowbar, he took down the ceiling in what was going to be David's bedroom. That's all he did. He took it down and closed the bedroom door and it stayed that way for two years. Then he started on the bathroom and toilet. Down came the walls that separated the bathroom from the toilet and landing. It took him three months to put up new ones. He did put in a new bathroom suite including a large shower, he even started tiling the walls, but then it stopped and we were left with holes in the floor boards, half tiled walls, no door and live wires poking from the wall *above the bath*! To this day my children still call out 'going to the loo' as a throwback to the lack of privacy from those chaotic days.

There was the time he bought four old dining chairs from an auction and stripped the paint from two of them. He half decorated the lounge but didn't put the carpet down. 'I've started so I'll finish' meant nothing to Bob.

So here I was, my home feeling as if it was falling down around me and next to nothing to live on.

I began to descend into a dark depression. Fear kept me awake at night, staring at the web I had created above me. During the day I put on a facade of contentment and coping, not wanting anyone to know how bad things were getting and how I was feeling. I was worried they would think I was a bad mother, or that I was simply feeling sorry for myself. And I worried that they would get tired of my neediness.

After the children had gone to bed, I started to drink, just a couple of glasses of wine to start with and I was rewarded with a blessed nights sleep. But of course it didn't stay like that. A couple of glasses grew to a bottle, then two bottles, then a litre and finally a litre and a half. I would convince myself that I had it under control. Because I couldn't afford to feed the children *and* myself, I fed the children only. Food for me was replaced with drink.

I felt I was coping. I still managed to wake up before the children and remove every sign of the web of protection but of course this couldn't last.

I vaguely remember a morning being woken by David. He had a mug of tea in his hand and was staring in wonder at the web above him.

"I've been trying to wake you mummy. I dressed Louise and made her some breakfast, she loved this," he said, staring again at the web. Louise appeared in the doorway, looking up and clapping her hands with glee at the wonder of the web. She threw herself on me then pulled away. "Eeeooooow!" she cried, wrinkling her tiny nose, "You smell like daddy."

Horrified, I crawled off the sofa and with some difficulty went upstairs to scrub my teeth and dress. My head was throbbing, I felt sick, and I couldn't focus.

I staggered back down the stairs, almost falling the last two, David reaching out his arms to try to save me. We left the house and I held their hands for the 5-minute walk to the school. The next thing I remember is the screech of breaks and I heard the children scream in fright. I had lead them across the road without looking and a car had narrowly missed mowing us down. The driver now sat gripping the steering wheel of his car, his head on his hands.

I remember Jayne was there with her two boys, she took the children's hands from mine.

"Go home Babs," she said, her eyes flashing anger at me. "Go home and sleep it off, I'll take Louise – pick David up later from school."

"Thanks", I mumbled weekly.

"I'm not doing it for you," she spat at me. Then looking at my pale-faced children she said, "I can't believe you are doing this after everything you and your kids have been through. Now go home I'll see you later."

She stormed off toward the school, other mothers stared at me, a mixture of sympathy and disgust on their faces.

I staggered home, went inside my house and locked the door. I raced up the stairs and threw up in the toilet, a disgusting smell of vomit and wine hitting me. I slipped down onto the floor, tears of the strain of heaving pouring down my face.

I sat there for at least an hour until the heaving subsided then, groping the walls to steady myself, found my way to Louise's bedroom and collapsed drunkenly onto her bed.

I awoke to the sound of banging on the back door, my head throbbed but at least the haze in front of my eyes had cleared. I rushed into the bathroom and threw cold water over my face. I glanced into the mirror, disgusted at the red eyes that stared back at me … 'what was I doing? What was I thinking of? I could have killed my children, I was no better than Bob'!

The banging on the door seemed to get louder and was now followed by "Babs, BABS, open this bloody door!!"

It was Kate and she was furious.

She paced up and down the kitchen …

"How could you?"

"Haven't they been through enough?"

"Just like bloody Bob."

"Thought better of you."

On and on she ranted, clearly shaken by what Jayne had almost certainly told her.

Then she grabbed hold of me and shook me like a child, the motion sending me fighting her in fright.

"Babs," she said now calmer, noticing the panic in my eyes, "Babs, calm down!"

"I'm sorry, I'm sorry, I'm sorry," I screamed back at her.

Kate put her arm around me and led me toward the lounge, glancing down at the floor, puzzled at the bits of rope and belts she saw lying there.

When we reached the lounge, she stared in confusion at what remained of my web.

"What the …… ?"

Her voice faded away as her eyes followed the web from the lounge to the dining room and back out to the front door. It was attached to every window, every door, and suddenly she knew what it was about.

"Oh Babs," she said, "Why didn't you tell me? I thought you were OK, coping, I didn't think, I should have known, I am so… so very sorry."

In silence we took down the web. I felt her watching me as I checked the doors and windows, making sure they were all closed and locked.

"You're not alone," she said, coming over to me, putting her arms around me, "I'm with you, we'll get through this together."

Kate took two weeks off work to be with me, or rather to keep an eye on me. We'd been best friends for only three years but it had always been one of those rare and very special friendships only women seem able to enjoy.

There were 18 years between us but this didn't affect our friendship, she being mature and crazy, me being immature and crazy!

We shared a love of music and sport, especially netball and badminton. Kate had started to play for my club when she was about 16, she was a great player, the other girls adored her and she was a valued member of the first team. Then suddenly she had vanished. Her friends said they knew she was in her flat but not answering the door. One admitted knowing Kate suffered from periods of depression. I took a chance and phoned her, she didn't say much but I knew she was listening.

"Look Kate," I had said, "Why don't you come and stay with us? You can have a room to yourself, play music, sleep all day, or be with us, it's entirely up to you."

An hour later she arrived on her bike, gorilla rucksack on her back, mostly packed with cassettes and sweets for the children and she stayed for about a month. She was one of those special people who knew instinctively how to talk and play with children and my two fell in love with her. Bob also liked having her around. It meant he could disappear for days on end knowing that Kate would be there for the children and me.

Kate and I recognised in each other kindred spirits. We could both be the life and soul of the party but had great periods of unexplained depression, when we would feel the need to separate ourselves from other people. We learned to recognise each other's moods, when to push and when to step back.

My periods of depression would make me feel very tired. Kate would leave me in the lounge to rest, take the children and a radio into the large kitchen and whilst she cooked a delicious meal I would hear the radio playing at top volume and she and the children would be rocking and rolling and singing along to the music, at the top of their voices. It never failed to bring me out of my melancholy.

It was a little more difficult for her, with her unexplained dark thoughts and memories, but the children and I always recognised a 'leave Kate alone' day. I knew one day she would tell me what troubled her.

Those two weeks helped to turn my life around. I quit the booze and the web of security didn't return.

She was there when Bob took to making drunken phone calls in the middle of the night, threatening me, accusing me of not giving him a second chance. A second chance could very easily have seen me dead!

She was there when he started to drive by the house and she was there when he parked across the road.

She was the one who phoned the police whilst I cowered in a corner but we were both there when the police arrived and dragged him away. Oh how we celebrated, with a Chinese takeaway and a large bottle of pop.

One of my fondest memories of those hard times was being packed off for the day by Kate and the children. They kept sniggering and nudging each other with an obvious shared secret. I needed the break, so off I went, to spend a day window-shopping in nearby Chelmsford.

Much as I loved my children, it was wonderful being on my own and not hearing the constant, 'can I have?', and 'mummy I need' followed by the obvious blackmail of 'everyone else has one.'

I drove home feeling relaxed and happy.

The children rushed to greet me as I came through the gate.

"You have to close your eyes mummy," David said, whilst Louise jumped up and down clapping her tiny hands.

Either side of me and holding my hands, the children led me into the house, then carefully up the stairs and in the direction of my bedroom. I wanted to pull back but their grip seemed to become more determined, as if they were expecting my reluctance to enter.

I heard the door open …

"Open your eyes mummy," said David softly, giving my hand a comforting squeeze.

"We did it, we did it, we did it!" squealed Louise, returning to her energetic, excited self. Jumping up and down she added, grinning from ear to ear, "Kate helped a little."

I looked into my bedroom, the scene of so many of my nightmares and the nightmares vanished!

Kate stood over by the window, smiling apprehensively.

The double bed had gone. In its place was a comfy-looking single bed, made up with Louise's Little Mermaid quilt cover and pillowcases.

The walls had been painted in a cheerful buttercup yellow and the ceiling was blue with tiny, silver stars painted on it. There were Little Mermaid curtains at the windows and cheerful, shell-covered bedside lamps.

The room was unrecognisable, nothing of my nightmare remained.

"A childish theme I know," said Kate, "But we were on a budget. Do you think you could make this your room again?" she asked, now really worried as the tears started to flow freely down my face.

"Oh yes," I almost whispered, looking around the cheerful room,

"Yes Kate, I most certainly can but only if …….
WE CAN *ALL* FIT ONTO THE BED!!!"

With that, the four of us threw ourselves onto the little bed, fighting over the quilt and pillows, screaming with laughter, uncaring when one of the legs gave way under the weight and strain.

And that, my friends, was one of the happiest days of my life!

THE BUSINNESS

For two years, Bob and I had run a small business from home. We sold charcoal to Indian Restaurants. Yes I know – how does anyone get into that? Well my father had worked as an accountant for a coal merchant in Ipswich. An Indian restaurant owner, having difficulty buying good quality charcoal for his tandoori ovens, had approached him for help. Although being presented with a good business plan by my father, his employers were reluctant to diversify. Knowing Bob and I were struggling financially, as always, he approached us with the plan. He suggested we consult a bank about financial backing and start selling charcoal ourselves. In the summer we could keep a small amount in the garden, and sell it domestically for barbeques.

Dad had already found a supplier in Portugal, had been there to see its preparation and quality. He had worked out a business plan and cash flow chart and had even found several interested buyers.

Bob, he suggested, would do all the heavy work, unloading the container when it arrived and deliver the charcoal. I would keep the books, canvass buyers throughout London and East Anglia, take the orders and plan the deliveries. I would also prepare a mail shot and advertise the charcoal for barbeques in the local shops and newspapers. Dad emphasised that as restaurants were only open at lunchtimes and evenings, this would not detract from my main role of home-keeper and mother.

I was thrilled with the plan. As much as I loved being a mother, I had never been comfortable with a life made up purely of domesticity. I loved working and God knows our family desperately needed *my* business acumen. It had often been claimed I could sell fridges to Eskimos and I had been a very successful 'story getter' as a journalist.

Within weeks, Bob, with the support of my father, had secured a loan by re-mortgaging our house. A netball friend who owned a farm rented us, at a very reasonable price, a dry barn to store the charcoal. We bought a frighteningly battered Luton van, which, Bob assured me, was 'up for the job'. Dad gave me a crash course on bookkeeping and with my gift of the gab we soon had over 100 customers.

With that, 'Anglia Charcoal' was up and running and with a handful of orders in his pocket, Bob went off to do our first deliveries. At first it all went extremely well, the money coming in each month was covering the cost of the charcoal, the rent and other expenses and very soon we started to make a tiny profit, barely enough to live on but I was already used to scrimping and saving.

It was a completely different story by the time we divorced. Bob had taken to drinking and gambling away the profit. He would fail to make deliveries and often left me in a panic, trying to find people to help me unload a container full of 12-kilo bags of charcoal.

It was therefore not difficult, following our divorce, to persuade the bank manager that I should be given the chance to run the business on my own. I thought I had blown it when the ever-present Louise managed to escape the constraints of her pushchair and with the strength that belied her 3-year-old body, pushed over a huge potted plant, the soil finding its way over and *into* his previously beautifully polished shoe. Unable to move, transfixed with horror and speculating whether or not his letter opener was sharp enough to slash my wrists, I watched in amazement as this incredibly handsome young man emptied the soil from his shoe, brushed as much as he could from his sock, hobbled over to Louise and picking her up, looked at my pulsating red face and said, "Oh please don't be embarrassed Mrs Cunningham, she's done me a favour, I always hated that plant!" He returned to his desk and holding her firmly on his knee (boy I wished that was me) he gave her pencils and paper and continued our discussion, only now and then removing her plump little fingers from his eyes, nose and ears, when the magic of the new toys no longer held her interest.

So I became the proprietor of 'Anglian Charcoal'. The simple use of an 'n' changing it from Anglia to Anglian, making it mine and nothing more to do with Bob Cunningham.

It was obvious from the start that I wouldn't be able to do the deliveries, the bags almost bigger than I was, although David did offer to give up school to help me.

"We can do it mummy, I think together we make a man," he had said solemnly one morning, as Louise and I walked him to school.

"It's OK sweetie," I said, smiling down at my sweet-natured little boy, "I'll sort something out."

So my first task as proprietor was to find a driver. Jen, one of my netball friends, who with Lou, another friend and player, ran Louise's Montessori nursery school in Halstead, had suggested I dropped Louise off at the nursery one morning and then trawl the local pubs, "You'll find plenty of men *not* looking for work there," she laughed.

To her and everyone else's surprise, considering my loathing of men and alcohol, I did exactly that. I dropped Louise off the next day and then went on a pub-crawl. In the very first pub I went into I asked the landlord if he knew of anyone looking for work as a driver.

"Nigel," he shouted out. "You're looking for work aren't you? This lady needs a driver".

"Yes mate," Nigel replied. I found myself looking into the gentle, inquisitive brown eyes of a great bear of a man with long dark curly hair, and thick unkempt beard and moustache.

"How much?" he asked.

Oh good Lord, catching on quick, I realised I had no idea of how much to pay a driver. Not prepared to throw a figure in the pot, I asked how much he was looking for.

YOU DON'T KNOW WHAT IT'S LIKE

"Tell you what," he said, in a surprisingly well-educated voice, as he pulled out a pen from his shirt pocket and started scribbling figures and words onto a beer mat, "You take a look at this, talk it over with your man, my phone number's on there – give me a call when you've decided. I can start as soon as you like."

I picked up the beer mat and tucked it into my bag. "There's no man," I corrected him, causing his bleary-eyed companion to give him a playful nudge, "I'll be in touch," I said, rising to leave. I put my hand out to him and tried miserably to return the grip as my small hand was completely swallowed up in his massive grasp.

As I left the pub I heard shouts of "Gooooooo Nige!" and "Wanna co-driver Nige?" followed by loud raucous laughter. All *I* could think was, 'I've got myself a driver! ... Goooooooooooo Babs'!!!!

That night, the children tucked up in bed, staring from Nigel's beer mat to my ledger, I thought I could just make the figure he was asking, if I could get at least another 10 good customers. Confident that was achievable, I phoned him.

"It's a deal," I said to him. "Can you come over tomorrow morning? We can go over the details and you can pick up the van. Oh and I need to see your driving licence," I suddenly remembered to add.

After Nigel agreed to come the next day, I hurriedly telephoned Kate to see if she was also free. I was reluctant to be alone in my house with a strange man. As ever, Kate promised to be there for me.

47

I made myself a cup of coffee and went back to my desk. I noticed it was 8 pm. 'No time to waste,' I thought, as I picked up the yellow pages, turning to *Restaurants – Indian* and started to canvass. By midnight I had 20 new customers and as I crawled exhausted up to my bed I thought again, 'Goooooooooooooooo BABS!!!'

THE BIG BOYS

Nigel and I made a good team. I quickly learned to trust him. He was hard working and reliable, never complained and dealt with all the problems the now, exhausted, old, unreliable Luton van threw at him.

He was a good salesman too. Staff in restaurants liked him and would often tell him where and when new restaurants were opening. Nigel would be the first at the door with a free bag of charcoal. He would negotiate a price and more often than not, they would become regular customers.

Nigel understood my situation completely: That I was a single mum struggling to run a business, I wasn't loaded with money and my children would always come first. The children loved him and after I had known him for a few months, I allowed David to go with him on a few deliveries, something his father always promised to do but like so many of his promises, he broke it. David would come home covered in coal dust, totally exhausted, deliriously happy, his faith restored in men. On one occasion – David still filthy dirty – Nigel took a photograph of the three of us sitting on the lawn in the back garden. "Perfect," he said smiling. "Perfect."

Gradually, between us, we were turning the business around and began to make a good profit. I was able to take a weeks' holiday, leaving the business in the capable hands of Nigel and returning to Mersea Island, burying our ghosts once and for all.

Little did we know that jealous eyes were monitoring our success. Other, much larger companies were eager to break into my area but so far my customers were staying loyal to me. They knew that if they under estimated their requirements, Nigel or I would happily drive to them with a couple of bags of charcoal, day or night, to keep them going – in my case, on occasions, with two children asleep in the back of the car.

Then my world fell apart. Nigel came to me one morning after the children had gone to school and told me he had to leave.
"I'm ill Babs, very ill. I have been diagnosed with motor neuron disease. I need to leave right away to be with my family in Somerset. They want me to be with them so they can look after me. I won't be able to look after myself for much longer. I'm so very, very sorry."
I was heartbroken, I opened my mouth but no words came out. I put my arms around this giant of a man, my head not even reaching his chin. He felt so strong. He freed himself and pushed me gently back onto my chair. He pulled up another, sat opposite me and took my hands in his.
"You are a wonderful woman Babs," he said, looking into my eyes, as I started to quietly cry, "I have learned to respect you so much over these

past months, respect you as a woman, as an employer, as a business woman, as a friend and as a mother. I have loved every back-breaking minute of working with you and I will never forget you and your beautiful children."

He got to his feet to leave, "Nigel … ", I said through the tears, shaking my head, groping for words, horrified at the lack of them, scared of using platitudes, "Nigel … I want … I need to say …"

He stopped me. "You don't need to say anything Babs, just let me go now and you must get on with the rest of your life." With that he walked away, turning once as he put the keys to the van on the table. "Kiss the children goodbye for me," he said, and with that he was gone.

It must have been 12 months later that I received a letter from a nurse at a Somerset Hospital, she wrote,

Dear Babs,
It is with enormous sorrow that I have to tell you that Nigel Hill died here, peacefully, a week ago. I want you to know Babs, that in the last six months I had loved Nigel deeply and although he tried to hide his feelings, I know he loved me too.
You and your children, Babs, had a special place in his heart and by his bed he had a photograph of the three of you, on the lawn of your garden. You all looked so happy but I often remarked on how dirty your son looked. It was sometime before he told me of a day he took the little boy with him on

a delivery and how your son had struggled to help him carry the heavy bags of charcoal. He said, if he had ever had a son he would have wanted him to be just like David!

I write to you because not only was I sure you would want to know of his death but also because I only ever knew him small and weak in a wheelchair and latterly in his hospital bed.

Can you tell me anything about him? Only his family visited him here, I long to know more about him, I miss him so much.

Your friend

Marianne xxx

My reply;

Dearest Marianne,

I am so very sorry to hear of Nigel's death but so happy to know he had found true love.

We adored him and the children were heartbroken when he left. I was too upset to even ask for an address I could contact him at.

He was a giant of man in reality and in our lives. He was hard working, popular and had a great sense of humour.

He gave me confidence to see my way through some very hard times and the strength to go on when he left.

Nigel restored my children's faith in men and I would have trusted him with their lives and mine.

We are all the better for knowing a man like him Marianne and I will never ever forget him.

YOU DON'T KNOW WHAT IT'S LIKE

Our love,
Babs, David, and Louise xxxx

I hoped my letter had been enough, for I never heard from her again.

Meanwhile, things went from bad to worse for Anglian Charcoal. The country was in the grip of a recession, restaurants were struggling, they would close overnight and re-open a few weeks later, with apparently a new owner. However, I would later discover that the owner would have become the manager and the manager the owner, therefore the business was still run by the same family under a different name.

My new driver, after only a week, stole my van. The following driver sold my charcoal to restaurants – telling me they had closed – telling them I was no longer the proprietor.

The big companies tightened their strangle hold on the market and undercut my prices by so much, I could no longer keep hold of my most loyal customers. Every weekend Kate and I would drive miles debt collecting, more often than not given cheques that would bounce, incurring more and more charges from the bank.

In the end, almost relieved, I threw in the towel, selling my last bags of charcoal for barbeques. In total I was owed £13,000 I had no hope of ever collecting and I was in debt to the tune of £120,000.

Oh well 'blood from a stone', sprung to mind.

DEVELOPING A POVERTY MENTALITY
Seeing the Light

We sat crossed legged on the floor, the children staring puzzled at the old familiar button box I placed in front of us. Louise glanced down at her buttoned cardigan, then at David's shirt. When my V necked sweater showed no buttons at all she went to say something, then decided to wait and see what happened next.

"Right," I said, removing the lid. "We are going to talk about money and pretend that each button is a £1."

I counted out 108 buttons, one for every pound I received for Income Support and Family Allowance.

The children wriggled impatiently.

"Right, we need £10 a week for gas, £10 for electricity and £10 for water". I counted out 30 buttons and put them in a serial bowl.

"Then there's £5 for the phone, David you count those. Louise you take £5 for car tax, £5 for insurance". Beginning to enjoy the game, she took her time selecting buttons she felt were the size of a pound coin – decided the colour was wrong and tried again. David and I smiled patiently at each other, "Girls," he said, shaking his head.

She finally made her selection and I told David to take out £8 for coal, £5 for kindling and a whopping £10 for petrol.

"David take £20 for shopping and Louise £10 for both your swimming lessons."

Slowly the children counted out the buttons, the small pile dwindling gradually.

"That leaves us £10 for things like birthdays and emergencies and treats."

David nodded, completely understanding the tight budget we were living on.

Louise looked at David, then at me, then down at the pile of buttons. She suddenly lent forward, picked up the button box and tipped the remaining contents onto the small pile.

"There you are mummy," she grinned. "We have more money for treats now!"

Oh well, back to the drawing board!

Money was a constant worry. Housing benefits did not take the size or the condition of the property in which you were living into account. This was a four bed roomed detached house built in the 1930's. All the rooms were large with high ceilings. The double-glazing was old and breaking down, the gas central heating inadequate. I worried about the roof. A couple of times, when the weather outside had been blowing up a storm, the door to the attic had blown open.

We still had sewerage occasionally seeping into the garden and the moss continued to grow healthily along the crack in the damp course outside the kitchen.

Although retaining a happy, cheerful persona in front of friends and family, I would lie awake for hours at night, worrying.

David was capable of getting through a pair of school trousers a week. Heaven knows what he got up to and even pleading with him to be careful, made no difference – the holes in the knees continued to appear. I became adept at repair work. Trousers became shorts or served to make patches. I thanked God for all those horrendous needlework classes at school, remembering Mrs Jones peering down at me over her huge bosom and saying, "Young lady, I have never had a failure in this subject, don't you be my first." She would be so proud of me now.

Louise just grew, up one week, out the next, then in again. Shoes were her thing – destroyed in one wearing on occasions – and although I watched her like a hawk I never actually caught the moment she put her shoes through the mincing machine.

Clothing was the least of my problems: Why is it light bulbs always seem to blow on the same day and the washing machine grinds to a halt at exactly, precisely, the same moment the refrigerator ceases its cheerful humming in the corner of the kitchen?

Oh and there's more: Why do windscreen wipers fail to work when it decides to rain for a week? The boiler stops working when the weather turns to freezing. The toilet won't flush when your lovely neighbours are on holiday. The car breaks down 10 miles from home and 20 minutes before the children come home from school. AND ... you tear your stockings just before you go out for the first time in months and the zip breaks in your one decent pair of trousers!!

I adopted a poverty mentality. For example, when I shopped for food I never took the children and I always used a basket. Children can emotionally blackmail you into buying things they want but don't need, or brands they recognise instead of cheaper ones.

Carrying a basket means you can only buy what you can carry, far less chance of buying too much or too big. I used to count everything in my basket as £1 an item – that way I always had change and was never embarrassed at the till. Well nearly never!

I literally learned 'to shop around'. I found all my friends had favourite supermarkets and I trained them into letting me know where there were offers and bargains and what 'buy one get one free' deals were around and my wonderful friends often did a 'buy one get one for Babs'!

In fact, we all found this exchange of information useful, making me feel less isolated.

Then there's training yourself to cut coupons out of magazines and newspapers – well in my case other people's magazines and newspapers, as I didn't buy them.

Most of our clothing came from charity shops and I let everyone know I was not too proud to accept second hand clothes. It was like Christmas in our house every time someone brought bin liners full of clothing around. My children rarely got 'new' but they often got 'new to them.'

However, I always insisted their shoes were new – or maybe worn just once or twice – and new underwear was important, not expensive, maybe bought in the sales, but new.

One thing I hated with a vengeance, was feeling helpless, needy. I mean a friend in need can rapidly become a pain in the arse. I was determined to learn how to 'fix' things or 'make-do.'

In the past, employers had used the pretty, young, naïve Babs, to get around angry or difficult customers or clients. I don't think it was just my looks – I did have a certain skill with people, a certain charm.

I looked at myself critically in the full length mirror on my bedroom wall, 'hmm not bad for 41, good figure, nice smile, bright blue eyes and long dark hair, you could even say attractive.'

Don't worry, I wasn't thinking of becoming 'a lady of the night.' But the time had come to put my womanly wiles to work for the children's and my benefit.

An idea was forming in my head. I needed to learn how to fix things and I needed to learn quickly. OK, I couldn't clear the blocked sewage pipes, YUK – *that* was most definitely a job for the men in overalls. I was darned sure, on the other hand, that there were repairs I *could* do. Those little repair jobs, the skill of which men kept as a closely guarded secret.

My friends and I sat together in my lounge, drinking wine and eating chocolates whilst we deviously hatched a plan. We decided that, whenever one of them needed repairs done and a 'man that does' was hired to do the job, I would be there, watching, pretending to write a shopping list or some such thing but furtively keeping notes. I would be girlie and flirtatious and say things like, "Oooh how clever" and "What do you call that bit?" and with fingers crossed behind my back, "If you didn't have that could you use something else in its place?" I might even throw in a couple of "My, aren't you strong(s)."

They roared with laughter when Kate suggested I wore a pink negligee and fluffy mules, and Mags suggested they have a whip round and buy me a curly blonde wig and a push up bra. I was shocked when they started throwing fivers on the table and relieved when Jayne said, "Who's going for some more wine and a Chinese takeaway?"

As I waved goodbye to them from my front door, I thought how lucky I was to have such great friends. For many years we had played together on and off the netball pitch, some of them I had watched grow up, coached them, put them forward for Essex and England trials but they always came back to play me. They came to me with their problems and I found time to listen, often holding them whilst they cried. They were my girls, my friends and as I lay in front of the dieing embers of my fire, I basked in the warm thoughts of their friendship.

YOU DON'T KNOW WHAT IT'S LIKE

We couldn't have dreamt how well our little plan would work out. I learned an elastic band could keep a microwave cooker going. Brushes could be replaced in washing machines, indeed in cars too but I never did find out where. The back of a tumble dryer can be vacuum cleaned and often dislodging fluff will make it work again.

We conjured a hasty second plan, when the men from the council came to look at the sewage pipes.
Several of the girls were there all giggly and gorgeous. They made a great show of hustling me off to bed feigning a migraine, something I had never suffered from but I think my groaning was convincing enough.
They later told me they had made sandwiches, tea and coffee that they took out into the garden, inviting the two, overjoyed men to join them. They then told them the well-rehearsed "Babs' story": Wonderful friend and mother, nasty evil ex husband, two small starving children, spending all day making their clothes.
Every now and then, one of the girls would come and 'check' on me – but it was in fact to give me a progress report – then return to the picnic on the back lawn, shaking her head in concern.
Then Kate came rushing up the stairs …
"Can you hear that?" she asked, grinning from ear to ear. I shook my head a little puzzled – I could in fact hear something but couldn't make it out.

She led me into the bathroom and quietly opened the windows, "Listen," she whispered …

"Another two poles should do it Fred," a man said.

"What is that Kate?" I asked.

"That" she said, "Is the sound of two happy men, with full tummies, clearing your drains, FOR FREE!!"

My hands flew to my mouth to stop the squeal that threatened to escape. "I can't believe it!" I chocked.

"Well believe this," said the grinning Kate. "Neet (Anita was the glamorous, leggie, member of the team) has got their private phone numbers, so you can phone them any time, if you have anymore problems."

With that we flew back into my bedroom, quietly closed the door, leapt face down onto my crippled bed and grabbing a pillow each covered our heads and scweamed and scweamed until we were nearly sick!"

THE SINS OF THE PARENTS ......

Some of the hardest times are when your children are hurting, or humiliated, because of the situation in which they unwittingly find themselves. Mine had suffered far too much for their tender years.

The Family Court had – in its infinite wisdom, protecting the rights of the father and oblivious to the rights of the children – granted Bob and I joint custody with care and control to me.

The Judge had asked Bob …

Is *she* a good mother?" cocking his head in my direction.

"She's alright!" Bob had replied.

Did he ask me if Bob was a good father? Did he hell!! Maybe just as well – for I would have ranted and raved until I was dragged off in irons to Holloway prison, thrown into a cell and left to reflect on my appalling behaviour.

The horror of this decision meant Bob could constantly question any decision of mine affecting the children. It gave him the right to see his children whenever and wherever he chose. He was still not allowed to come within three miles of me, of course, but nonsense was made of that as – no surprise to me – Bob had recently lost his driving licence as a result of a drink/driving conviction and it was up to me to get the children to him.

The worse thing, however, and the thing that would fight for my attention during those long sleepless nights, was that if anything happened to me, the children would automatically be taken to their father. If ever I needed a reason to stay alive and stay healthy, it was that!

So some power over me was returned to my ex husband – and did he enjoy it! He questioned *everything* – their diet, their clothing, their friends, my friends – simply everything!

To start with, he insisted on having them every weekend, but I soon discovered that he often left them with other people whilst he went out for hours on end and they hardly saw him.

I would pick up two, grubby little strangers on a Sunday evening, their clothes thrown back into their bags, dirty and smelling. The journeys from Ilford back to Braintree were often in silence and instinctively, I knew not to question them about their father.

When we got home, the three of us would climb naked into a hot bath full of bubbles and toys and we would play until the water turned cold and my little people were once again back to their wonderful, happy selves.

Later one night, the bath time fun over, tucking Louise into her bed and kissing her now sweet smelling rosy cheek, she turned her blue eyes, so much like mine, to me and said,

"I don't really like the daddy".

"Don't you darling, why is that?" I asked her, worried.

"He smells," she said, "And he smokes funny smelling cigarettes and gets silly."

As I struggled to find something to say, she suddenly reached out her hand and touched my

breast and lifting her own pyjama top she said, "Look mummy, mine are all weared out."
With that, the daddy was forgotten. I pulled her to me and we laughed and laughed and I said, "Don't worry darling, I'm sure they will grow back."

I was worried about David, he so desperately wanted to support me, he wanted to be a man, to do things he felt men would do and he was still only 8 years old.
He so loved his father and his memories confused and haunted him. He didn't want me to miss having a man around. He also wanted me to know that not all men were going to hurt me.
I knew things had come to a head when Louise came to me in my bedroom one day and asked if she could do something or the other. When I refused she started to wail,
"But David said I could, you ask him, he said he's the daddy now," she cried.
David appeared at my bedroom door.
"Be quiet, Louise," he said, "And do as your mother tells you."
Oh boy, something had to be done.

I arranged for Kate to have Louise for the day and David and I climbed into my battered, rusty old BMW, to spend a day of fun together.
The BMW had been a 40th birthday present from Bob. He had asked what I had wanted and I'd replied, joking, "a microwave cooker and a BMW."
Well I got them both, the serial number beaten off

the microwave and the BMW towed home because it didn't have a gearbox!!

Within a week the car was on the road. He'd actually put in a new gearbox but I was haunted by a vision of a BMW parked somewhere, the bonnet forced open and the gearbox missing.

I'm not saying my ex husband was a 'tea leaf' but I have this fond memory of a phone call from my innocent mother, asking me to relay a message to him.

"Please tell Bob," she had said, "I would like to take him up on his offer. Next time he sees 'one of those lorries,' I would love a terracotta planter."

Oh dear, I could remember my mother asking Bob where he had got my microwave from, as it was extraordinarily large. He had replied, tapping the side of his nose with his index finger, "Off the back of a lorry, Helena. Any time you need anything, just phone me."

David sat excitedly next to me in the car, his imaginary steering wheel in his hands, changing the imaginary gears and making car noises rivalling those made by the tired old engine of my BMW.

By way of distraction, I got him to choose a cassette to play and we finished the rest of the journey rocking and rolling and singing our heads off to 'Status Quo.'

We had a wonderful day together in Castle Park, in Colchester. We kicked a ball around and then he played in the childrens' area on the swings, slides and roundabouts. I watched him dashing around from one piece of equipment to another, rallying other children to join him, his beautiful red hair shining in the sunlight.

Then we sat down on a blanket to have our picnic. I looked at his precious face. He had an explosion of freckles on his cheeks and his round hazel eyes were full of laughter as raspberry jam dripped down his chin. YES JAM!! Don't tell his father, this was David's day.

Whilst we ate we chatted about school and swimming and about Kate and the girls. We talked about Louise and the funny things she said and did and we talked about daddy.

David's eyes clouded.

"Do you miss him?" I asked gently.

"Yes," he said, looking at me, worried he would hurt my feelings.

"Do you?" he asked.

It was one of those moments I wanted to lie to my son but I had made up my mind never to lie to my children. So a variation of the truth was required.

"Sometimes," I said. "Sometimes I miss him, or I miss the man he used to be, do you understand what I mean by that?"

"Yes," he replied sadly. "When he used to come home and play with me and make you laugh. When he used to come home with stuff and you would say 'get that thing out of my house'" he laughed.

I recalled the occasion David was referring to. The children and I had been sitting at the kitchen table playing snap. Louise was winning because she just kept saying 'snap, snap, snap, snap,' – say it enough times you are bound to get it right!

The door flew open and there stood Bob, his face red with exertion, grinning from ear to ear, propping up a huge, ugly fruit machine.

"Get that thing out of my house!" I had shouted at him.

"But it could be full of money," he argued.

"I don't care if it's got the Queen's jewels in it, get it out!!!"

David had run to help his father and the fruit machine was banished to the garden shed and there it stayed until we divorced, surprisingly not one of the things Bob had wanted to take with him. Eventually, I got a fiver for it, from the Rag and Bone man. "It might be full of money," I said.

"Yeah right missus," the ruddy faced man had replied.

"David," I said cautiously, "He will always be your daddy, what happened between us had nothing to do with you or Louise. He will always love you," I added, trying to keep the doubt out of my voice.

"But he hurt you," said David, suddenly bursting into tears. "He hurt your face and made it all bloody and I didn't save you. I have to look after you and Lou now."

I grabbed my sweet boy to me as his body was wracked with sobbing. I stroked his hair and kissed his wet face, gently rocking him in the safety of my lap.

YOU DON'T KNOW WHAT IT'S LIKE

"You couldn't have done anything my sweet, you were so tiny. If anything you *did* stop him when you brought us the milk."

"But mummy he hurt you, he hurt you so badly!" David sobbed, "And he told me it was all your fault."

"No one deserves that David," I said to him gently. "Whatever they have done, hitting people is not the answer."

"David, you don't have to look after Lou and me, that's my job. It's your job to show me that I am getting it right by being the best, the happiest little boy I know. If I'm getting it wrong, I will know. Whenever you need to talk to me you tell me and we will find more days like this to spend together, just the two of us."

I put my hand under his chin and gently raised his face to look at me. His eyes, red and swollen from the tears, had thankfully lost some of the fear they had shown for so many months and were now heavy with exhaustion.

I continued to gently rock him in my arms and I hoped he had heard my last words as he gave in to sleep ... "I love you and Lou more than life itself, my son, my precious, precious son."

As the sun went down and the air grew cold, I carried him to the car. He didn't stir as I strapped him into his seat, he didn't stir when I carried him from the car into the house, he didn't stir when I undressed and put him to bed. My son slept the sleep of an innocent, my little boy had returned to me.

An hour later, Kate carried a sleeping Louise into the house and, so like her brother, she didn't wake as Kate put her to bed. We sat in the lounge later, talking about our day.

"I'm so scared I'm going to let them down Kate," I said solemnly.

"Let them down" she replied, incredulity in her voice. "Don't you know your children are a credit to you? After everything they have been through they are still polite and kind and extrovert and funny – you are getting it so right, *girlfriend*. Now about my wages …" she added, mischievously.

I was a 'Single Mother', my children were part of a 'Single Parent Family' and boy were we singled out. I stormed down the road to my son's school – a crumpled letter I had found in David's pocked, clutched in my hand.

I stood at the back of the hall and joined in as the children sang 'All things bright and beautiful, all creatures great and small, all things wise and wonderful, the Lord God made them all.' Yes, I thought angrily, even the children from Single Parent Families!!

When the hymn had finished and they sat down on the wooden floor, some of the children peered round at me inquisitively. I spotted the worried face of my son and smiled at him reassuringly. Not fooled by the rigour like grin on my face and knowing me far too well, he shrugged in quiet resolution and turned his face back to the figure on the stage. The headmaster, too, had spotted me and yes, I think some of the blood had drained from *his* face.

He and I had locked horns on several occasions and one look at my face warned him he was in for another battle. As the children filed quietly from the hall, Mr O'Donnell joined me and taking me by the elbow led me into his office.

"How can I help Ms Cunningham?" He asked.
"You can explain this," I said, placing the letter in front of him, making a great show of smoothing it out as much as I could.

He read aloud:

To the parents/guardian of <u>David Cunningham</u>   As your son/daughter will not be attending the four day educational trip to <u>Shugborough Hall, Staffordshire</u> he/she will be expected to write a short essay on <u>Where I went on my holiday last summer.</u>

Iain O'Donnell
Headmaster

"Yes," he sighed, "I do recognise it. Is there a problem?"
"Oh yes," I said, "I think there most certainly *is* a problem. First, what trip to Shugborough Hall?"

"Every child was given a letter to give to their parents about the £50 trip to Shugborough," he informed me.

"A letter in an envelope?" I asked.

"Eh no," he replied, "Just folded, we do try to save money on envelopes. There was nothing confidential in the communication."

"My son," I said slowly, deliberately, "Will have read this non confidential communication. He will have noted the £50 cost of the trip, he will have known that there was no chance of my getting that money together and he will have thrown the letter away before I even got sight of it."

"Not my problem Ms Cunningham," he said, arms behind his head, leaning back in his comfortable chair. "Your son should have known not to throw away a letter to his parents."

Ignoring the 'parents' jibe – he knew very well I was on my own – I rose slowly to my feet and said,

"It *will* be your problem Mr O'Donnell" – I smiled as sweetly as I could – "It will most certainly be your problem when I muster every placard waving, single parent I can to wave goodbye to the *rich kids* going on their four day educational trip to Shugborough Hall, and I will make sure the press have a wonderful photo opportunity to take pictures of the *poorer kids*, sitting on the grass verge outside OUR school, writing essays on imaginary holidays their PARENTS couldn't afford for them to go on!!"

I emphasised this last point by slamming my fist on his large expensive desk and turned to leave.

YOU DON'T KNOW WHAT IT'S LIKE

"Mrs Cunningham, what on earth do you expect me to do, where do you think I can get the money to pay for the children who can't afford the trip?"

"Bring and buy sales, rummage sales, raffle tickets, concerts, fines on late library books, a swear box in the staff room … and sell that dam desk.   I'll help, *all* the 'single parents' will help. Stop being complacent! Think about it whilst I go home to make my placard and when you want me, give a note to my son." And with that I turned and marched out of his office!

Six months later, Louise, Kate and I waved a tearful goodbye to David and the other children setting off for Staffordshire.   Amongst his clothes he would later find little notes and poems from Lou and me telling him we loved him … to remember to brush his teeth … to not eat too much chocolate … to write to us and, something I always said to my children … to Be Safe!

I glanced to my left and spotted Mr O'Donnell looking at me with a smile on his face. He put his hands together in silent applause, then turned and went back into the school.

This was one of many times I fought for the rights of children from poorer families.

When the price of swimming lessons rose to a cost well out of my reach, I stood outside the pool entrance, where a large sign read: EVERY CHILD SHOULD LEARN TO SWIM and held up my own placard saying: BUT IF YOU CAN'T AFFORD IT THEY WILL HAVE TO DROWN! Within 24 hours the charge for children from families living on benefits returned to the original price.

I fought for all children to be given their luncheon vouchers every Monday *in class*, rather than the children on free school meals being called to the school office to collect their vouchers. I ran a second-hand school uniform shop once a month in the school hall. I held fundraising events that would benefit all children and I became the oracle on benefits and grants available for single parents.

It is truly amazing what one person can achieve if they have fire in their hearts, determination and a really bad temper!!!

BREAKING THE NEWS TO MUM AND DAD

The time had come to see my parents and up-date them on the massive changes in my life. For many years my relationship with my parents had been tenuous and they were never the first people I would turn to in times of trouble. I loved them both dearly but just failed to find common ground on which to communicate with them. I understand them now but as a child and in my teens and 20's I felt lonely and isolated, the odd one out, which in many ways I was.

My beautiful petite mother, who had long thick black hair and dark brown eyes, was of mixed race. She was brought up in India by her Indian mother and her English father. She had met my father in India during the war when he was serving there with the West African Frontier Force.

She was only 18 years old, naïve and innocent, whereas he was a 23-year-old man of the world having already enjoyed several 'full on' relationships. Apart from her obvious sultry beauty, my father fell in love with her innocence, her lack of guile and – as he once wrote in a letter home to his mother – her beautiful set of teeth!
They came from very different backgrounds. My mother enjoyed all the trappings of a wealthy family in India, nice home, servants and private education. My father, on the other hand, was born into a working class – or rather *hard working* – family. His mother was in 'service' and his father

worked the land. My father was a scholar, the first from his family to go to grammar school. It meant a 3 mile walk to and from school every day and he worked on a farm before and after school as well – wow – great respect Dad!

They were married within 12 months and very soon my mother found herself on board a ship on her way to England, with a new husband and baby girl – my oldest sister Lesley – and already pregnant with my brother David. How excited but scared she must have been.

I was quite a surprise to both my parents. Both Lesley and David were born with olive skins, dark brown eyes and black hair. I, on the other hand, was fair skinned with blonde hair and blue eyes. My mother often tells the tail of how she was convinced she had been given the wrong baby and had insisted on looking at all the other new babies in the maternity wing of the hospital, finally accepting that I was indeed hers. My father, who also had black hair and brown eyes, would tell me I was a throw back on his side of the family. He had a blonde-haired blue-eyed aunt.
I never met my maternal grand parents and have no memory of my paternal grandfather but my father's mother, I knew, disliked me. Although she lavished love, affection and attention on my brother and two sisters – for six years after me, my sister Jane was born – my grandmother often told me I was different and didn't belong and would push me away from her!

So I grew up with a feeling of not belonging, in the shadow of two stunningly beautiful sisters.

I'm not saying I was a 'dog', in fact I was quite attractive, but boyfriends would almost trip over their tongues when they met my sisters!

OK, so I didn't have the looks, but in my fight for attention I developed whit and humour all packaged together with a strong personality.

Unfortunately, some would say, I also developed a pretty rebellious nature, often putting me at odds with my frustrated parents.

I left home at 17 and worked as a trainee journalist on a Colchester newspaper. Away from the rigours of a strict and controlled upbringing, this newfound independency went to my head. In no way was I out of control. I didn't smoke, drank little alcohol and I would certainly never have entertained drugs but maybe, just maybe, my priorities were a little confused in the planning.

Away from my sisters, men saw me as extremely attractive and great company, quite a catch with intelligence thrown in. And there were plenty of young men in my world as journalism was still very much a man's world. In fact there was a whole police station full of young single men vying for my attention, so why oh why did my first love have to be a man newly separated from his wife, 8 years my senior?

Ken was a 26 year old handsome, hardened detective and although I tried to avoid him – at just turned 18 I was a little afraid of such an 'old' man's attention – he soon won me over.

My parents were horrified and within 24 hours of meeting him, severely told me they didn't want to see me again until the relationship with Ken was over! *That* took 4 long years and important occasions like their silver wedding anniversary – when they sent me back their present and card – and my 21st birthday – when I didn't receive a present or card – were lost to us forever.

During that time I also developed Glandular Fever and by the time I was on the road to recovery I weighed only 6 stone.

I was ill for six months and although they knew, I heard nothing from my parents. My flat mates looked after me, washed and gave me bed baths – with such a high fever I was oblivious to my surroundings. They fed and nurtured me through my recovery and they gave me emotional support when the sorrow of isolation from my family threatened to engulf me.

I think it was then that I first began to draw away from my family turning more towards my friends, who seemed always to be there for me.

My relationship with Ken eventually ran its course. He had wanted me to move in with him but this really did go against the grain, this to me was 'living in sin' something I just couldn't do – well this *was* the late 60's and the madness hadn't quite reached my doorstep! He eventually started to have affairs, finally – unknown to me until told by a very concerned friend – setting up home with another girl in a nearby town.

YOU DON'T KNOW WHAT IT'S LIKE

I was heartbroken and unable to work. My worried editor rushed me back to my parents' home, thus giving them their first 'I told you so' opportunity.
Within 7 days I was transferred to the Brentwood edition of the newspaper – people who cared about me eager to put as many miles as possible between Ken and me.

All this was running through my head as I drove through the beautiful countryside to my parents' bungalow in Suffolk. Although my parents adored my children, I had decided to leave them in the capable hands of Kate. If our conversation turned 'pear shape' I didn't want my children to be there when I blew!!
I had already decided to play down Bob's violence as it would be far too difficult and painful for either of my parents to comprehend.
They greeted me with open arms but with the usual,
"We never see you and our grandchildren" and "Have you put on weight?" followed by "Do you think your hair suits you like this?" My mother always preferred my hair short and in my life there had been many styles and colours. Recently I had gone red and my hair was long and curly, my son had complained he was the only redhead in the family, so whilst it was important to him, I decided to join him. Needless to say, he was thrilled.

It was a lot for my parents to take in …
I had left Bob and we were now divorced.

The business had failed and I was now living on benefits.

Yes, the children were well and happy … I was still living in Braintree … I saw a lot of Kate … I still played netball and badminton and yes I *did* have time.

No, I didn't have another man in my life … and no I *didn't* need a man!

On and on it went starting with serious and rapidly turning to trivial.

"Oh well Barbara," … Oh dear, here we go … only my parents called me Barbara and usually a lecture followed ….

"We did try to warn you about Bob. I hope you are not letting him see those two beautiful children, they are, after all, the only thing you've got right in your life!"

I put my hand to the back of my neck as my hackles fought to rise, fighting against the weight of the rest of the hair on my head.

"The Family Court gave us joint custody," I started to say …

"Yes but you're not letting him see them are you?" my mother persisted.

"I have no choice," I replied.

"Choice, choice, there's always choice, I don't think you should allow him to see those children," my mother continued.

I turned to my father for support but none was forthcoming, he rarely took my mother on when she was on a mission.

"Besides," I foolishly added, "They want to see their father and his family ..."

Big, big mistake!

"You must *not* let those children see him," my mother insisted, getting quite cross, "And as for that family, well you know how I feel about them!!"

My mother had never quite recovered from an incident that occurred at David's christening. My brother-in-law, Harry, had come out of the bathroom with a tampon held up to his mouth and had asked my mother for a light. She was horribly embarrassed and this was added to when Bob's complete family roared with laughter, enjoying her confusion.

"They are such a rough lot", she continued, her eyes filling with tears and I was able to remain calm because I knew her anger came out of love and protection toward David and Lou.

"I'll do my best mum," I said to placate her.

She wiped her eyes with a crisp little handkerchief she took from her sleeve. She had to be the only person I knew who didn't use tissues.

"Do you want some cake"? she asked. "I'll get you a slice of my cake, I know you can never resist fattening food." Another famous swipe!

Alone together, my father at last, broke his silence.

"He hurt you didn't he?" he asked.

In a way, my father and I were close, maybe because I was the only one who resembled his side of the family, who shared his quick wit and sense of humour. Or maybe because I had followed him into the world of newspapers, although he hadn't been a journalist, only dabbling sometimes, covering local football ties.

He had been the Managing Director of a large series of newspapers, having started at the bottom selling small adds but with a steady and gradual rise to the top.

He had resigned his position when the series was taken over by one of the large powerful nationals. The London directors constantly undermined him at board meetings and colleagues he had worked with for many years, men he knew and respected, were losing their jobs.

"Yes dad, he hurt me badly," I replied and he knew I wasn't talking emotions.

"Are you OK now?" he asked solemnly.

"I come from strong stock dad, I'm doing OK," I replied, trying to smile reassuringly.

"You know, your mother is right, the children should not see him but I do understand it's out of your hands."

"Try explaining that to mum," I begged.

"No," he smiled, "more than my life's worth. Let's just eat cake and get fat."

I drove away with no promises of support, financial or otherwise. I had told them I was now on Income Support and how much that was but it fell on deaf ears.

However, I did have the remains of the yummy coffee walnut cake, wrapped up in foil, sitting on the car seat next to me, so not a complete waste of a journey.

A MAN IN MY LIFE

'She's up to something,' I decided, as I put down the phone. I had just finished a long conversation with Neet, the glamorous, blonde, leggie member of our crowd.

"You *must* come and see me," she had insisted, "I'm working in 'The Drury' in Colchester, Layer Road, do you know it, it's where the football ground is, the 'U's', you must know it?"

Yes I knew it, from my newspaper days, one of those pubs that came under the heading of 'Beware, this pub is full of drunken squaddies.'

She scoffed at me when I told her this.

"That was bloody years ago," she said. "It's not like that now. Anyway, they are all away in Kuwait or Saudi or somewhere hot with sand and oil. You must come and see me, bring Kate and the others."

Anita and I had been friends for over two years. I first spotted her at a summer netball rally, playing goal shooter for a Colchester team. She was a brilliant player, loud and gobby, the air turning blue with her expletives, but I couldn't help laughing as I watched her play. Most of her frustration was aimed at her own team. She knew damn well that if they would just get the ball to her she would reward them by putting it in the net.

She looked over and noticed me watching her. I was well-known in the world of netball, had been around for years. I ran a large successful club, I coached and umpired to County level and I was the press officer for the Essex Netball League.

Shrugging her shoulders, her palms raised in the air, she shouted across to me, "Wanna goal shooter?"

After the game, I drew her away from her team.

"If you are serious," I said, "I would love you to join us. I'm going to need a goal shooter, Kelly's moving away."

"The thing is," I added, "You would be on a month's trial, so don't burn your boat with your team. It's really important to us that any new member is not just a great player – she would have to fit in too. We are great friends on and off the court and we don't take on prima donnas. And it *is* 'we'. I make the final decision but only after all the girls have had their say. So what do you say"?

A week later, Neet played her first game for Anglian Charcoal. The business had gone but we just couldn't come up with a new name for the team and were too well known as Anglian Charcoal to be bothered to try. She didn't drive, so I got to know her really well, picking her up from Colchester after she had finished work and taking her back to mine before a match. She fell in love with my children and they adored her.

So when I got the phone call telling me I had to go to this pub to see her, I recognised urgency in her voice, but decided she was probably trying to find me a cash in hand job and thought no more of it.

Kate and I stood at the bar of The Drury. I looked around nervously, still sporting my fear of drunken men. I needn't have worried, the soldiers were indeed away – there wasn't a uniform in sight –

and the ever-protective Kate, I knew, would see anyone off who came too close.

We watched Neet, the perfect barmaid, smiling sweetly and chatting away to the handful of men at the bar, each one of them, I'm sure, convinced her beautiful smile was just for them. She was thrilled to see us, stretching across the bar to give us both a hug. She took our order and glided back to the other end of the bar.

I was alarmed, however, when I heard her say to someone I couldn't quite see,

"Jim, JIM, she's here! Look, that's her at the other end of the bar, the short one with the big hair, that's Babs."

'Cheek,' I thought, trying to tame my unruly mop. Nothing I could do about my 5' 1" – 'more depth than height,' I was once told by a 6' 2" DSI.

The owner of the name 'Jim' – a tall, well-built man with what I guessed was prematurely grey hair, as he had thick black eyebrows – stepped back from his companions and looked at me curiously. He then said something to Neet, which can't have been bad, as her response was,

"Yeah – see, told you she was gorgeous!"

"Hey you two," called Neet, beckoning. "Come this end so I can talk to you."

As I went to say 'Its OK, we are fine where we are', Kate picked up my bag and with purpose took hold of my elbow, pulling me toward the group of men at the other end of the bar and planting me next to Jim. She and Neet exchanged a wink and I thought 'Oh my God, I've been suckered, Kate's in on the plot.' I glared at both of them but got angelic little smiles in return.

"Jim Stewart," said the handsome man, putting his hand out toward me, a look of amusement in his brown eyes.

"Loved your last film," I quipped, returning his firm handshake.

"Sorry?" he said, looking confused.

"Don't apologise," I retorted, "Probably not your fault." Once again I glared at Kate who dismissed my look and said to Neet,

"You did warn him didn't you?"

"Didn't bother, if he can't handle her, we've wasted our time" she laughed, ignoring my angry stare.

For the next hour or more, Jim, a Staff Sergeant with the Royal Signals, tried desperately hard to make conversation, getting sarcasm and nonchalance in return. To his credit, he ploughed on regardless and eventually I started to warm to his friendly Lancashire accent and his steady, admiring gaze.

I couldn't resist asking him questions, the journalist in me ever present. He answered every question, telling me he was 46, he was from Bolton, had been in the army for over 20 years and was due to retire, if he didn't take promotion, in four years.

He was divorced and had two young daughters who lived with their mother in Bolton. Jim had been stationed in Colchester for just four months and managed the officers' mess at nearby Goojerat Barracks.

I was impressed with the respect the young soldiers who drifted into the pub showed him, calling him Sir and being gently corrected.

"Staff," said Jim.

"Staff Sir, yes Sir, sorry Sir," said one young man, blushing to the roots of his well-groomed hair. He didn't look old enough to be out of school let alone in the army.

Jim laughed as he turned back to me, catching the smile on my face.

"You're very pretty when you smile, Babs," he said.

Oh my God, time to go, I thought.

"Kate, we're out of here, babysitters remember?"

Kate, who had been happily chatting with Neet and a tiny little guy, looked puzzled and went to say something.

"Now!" I said.

We both hugged Neet and left the bar. Jim followed us out and called to me.

"Can I ring you Babs, what's your phone number?"

I shouted my number at him and climbed into the passenger seat of Kate's rusty little Ford.

"He'll never remember that," I laughed.

"You don't have a babysitter," said Kate, dismissing my previous comment. "The children are at *the daddy's*."

"I know," I replied laughing, "clever aren't I?"

"Well I wrote my number down for Pete," she said.

"Who's Pete?"

"The guy talking to Neet and me," she replied. "He was nice … funny."

With that we drove back to Braintree in silence, both lost in our separate thoughts of the evening.

Two days later, I returned home after picking David up from school, to find a message on my answer phone.

"Hi Babs, Jim Stewart here, bet you didn't think I would remember your phone number! Anyway, I would really like to see you again. I'll phone back later for a chat. I hate these infernal answering machines."

With that he was gone, 'well I'm not going to speak to you,' I thought to myself.

I should have said something to my son, for an hour later he called upstairs to me.

"Mummy, a man on the phone for you, says he's Jim from the other night. I'll leave the phone at the bottom of the stairs."

With that I heard him run outside shouting to Lou to stop playing with the coal. 'Still the daddy' I thought, walking reluctantly down the stairs and picking up the phone as if it were going to bite me.

"Hi Jim," I said, anxiously.

"Hello Babs, glad your little boy answered," he laughed.

'Damn him,' I thought, he knew I wouldn't have answered if I'd heard his voice on the answer phone.

"Look," he said, not giving me a chance to reply, "I'm not working Friday night, would love to see you, say 8 o'clock, in The Drury, or would you like me to come to Braintree?"

"No, don't come here," I replied hastily, too hastily, I hadn't given my brain time to catch up with my mouth as I heard myself say, "I'll come there."

"Great," he said, sounding surprised, "I'll see you then, looking forward to it, bye." And he was gone before I had a chance to change my mind.

Damn, damn, damn!!!

So it was a few days later that I found myself getting ready for my first 'date' in 14 years. I felt sick with nerves. Downstairs I could hear the noise of the children playing with my babysitters for the night, Kate and Pete. This was the second time I had met Pete. Kate had brought him round to meet the children and me on the evening of their first date and here they had stayed – playing music and dancing with the children, playing chase and hide and seek. I liked him instantly and it was if they had known each other all their lives, showing no signs of awkwardness or discomfort in each other's company.

As I entered the lounge, all four faces turned and stared at me – David the first one to break the silence.

"Wow mummy, you look beautiful!"

"Like a princess," said Lou.

"Lucky man," Pete commented smiling and nodding.

"Not too short?" I asked, bear legged, knees together, wiggling in my high heels and pulling at the hem of my tight little black dress, trying to make it longer. I was still very slim, struggling to gain weight after months of not being able to eat anything substantial without feeling sick.

My hair, short and spiky, was now light brown with blonde highlights, having been restyled that morning by Shirley, a hairdresser and netball playing friend, who had often said she couldn't wait to get her hands on my unruly hair.

"Babs, you look stunning," said Kate, smiling at me. "You're going to do his head in," she laughed.

"I really don't want to go," my eyes were stinging with held back tears.

"Get out of here! I doubt he will be there, you're going to be an hour late." Kate thrust my bag and car keys at me.

"You'll have a great time and so will we, the second you drive down the road!"

As I drove past the house, I saw David and Louise standing on the windowsill, held there safely by Pete and Kate, waving and smiling and I wondered if it had really sunk into my children's heads, that I was going to meet another man, a man who wasn't 'the daddy'.

Jim was still there. Having phoned my home and ascertained I was on my way, he had made the wise decision to sit at a table in the garden of the pub, where he could keep an eye on the car park. Just as well, as I doubt my shaking legs would have carried me through the door. He pecked me on the cheek and linked my arm in his.

"Would you like to go in, or sit out here?" he asked. "It's packed inside, some of the lads are celebrating being home from Kuwait."

"Out here," I said relieved, not sure I could cope with the noise I could hear coming from inside the busy pub.

On the table was a half drunk pint of beer and a glass of wine with a beer mat covering the top.

"I've been drinking slowly," he smiled, as if to reassure me this wasn't his second or third pint. I later discovered that Anita had told him a little about Bob and his problem with drink, without going into too much detail, and this kind man had taken it into consideration and that pint was all he drank.

Once I had relaxed we got on extremely well and I allowed a little of my personality to show. I laughed and teased him about my experiences with the army, telling him how the Durham Light Infantry had taken over Colchester in the late 60's, when they had been posted to the town, leaving chaos in their wake

At one point, Jim got hold of both my hands and said,

"Do you realise what a beautiful woman you are, Babs?"

At that moment a large group of soldiers spilled out of the pub, laughing and swearing, throwing beer and crisps at each other. I felt myself freeze and pulled my hands from Jims.

He excused himself, got up from the table and with hands behind his back, walked slowly over to the group.

"Now then lads," he said in a loud purposeful voice. "Gather round," he added, when he had their attention.

Immediately they drew close to him, backs rigid, hands by their sides.

I couldn't hear what he was saying but I heard *them*.

"Sir, yes Sir, no Sir, sorry Staff, yes Staff."

To my horror he led them towards me.

"My lads would like to say something to you Babs," Jim smiled at me reassuringly.

One by one, he introduced all 20 of them to me, remembering their names and rank – even those of the few not in uniform – and one by one, wiping their hands on the side of their trousers, they shook my hand gently and apologised for the noise and their bad language.

To Jim's amazement I invited them to join us and even more amazingly, they did exactly that, dragging heavy tables across the lawn.

They vied for my attention and flirted with me and I loved every minute of their company, all fear a distant memory, and when more of their comrades fell out of the pub, they asked Jim if they could also join us. He sat with a smile on his face as I laughed and joked with these lovely young men, eventually telling them to 'clear off, as I was his.'

"Keep your head down boys," I laughed as one by one they kissed my cheek and the jovial crowd walked slowly back to camp, some wisecracking

that *when* I got bored with Staff, or fancied a younger man, they were available.   A few even gave me their telephone numbers and addresses.
As they disappeared from sight, I gave the pieces of paper to Jim and said,
"I won't need these."
Getting up, he walked around to my side of the table, pulled me to my feet, put his arms around me and kissed me.   Once again my legs felt weak!!

JIM

I looked out of the window at David and Louise, their little suitcases on the ground beside them, standing on the path on the corner of the road, waiting patiently for the daddy to pick them up.
They had been there for an hour and I had been in and out trying to persuade them to wait inside but they wanted to see daddy's new car coming down the road. They wanted to wave to him and I think, in David's case, he wanted to keep daddy away from mummy.

I knew he wasn't going to turn up. A car meant he could trawl the pubs of Essex, visit old friends and forget he had children.
I picked up the telephone and dialled Jim's number. He had been asking to meet the children but thus far I had refused, reluctant to bring a man into their lives. Now I decided today was the day.
Jim and I had had several dates. He had taken me to the Sergeants' Mess on camp and had introduced me to his friends – that in itself a big step for him – for he was a proud man and needed to feel right about me being introduced into his world – to know that I would at least *try* to stick with the protocols, many of them steeped in tradition.
It was the protocols he was most concerned about, for he realised I was a fiercely independent woman who wouldn't suffer fools, or foolish rules and regulations. But I accepted that this was Jim's

world – a world into which I soon became a welcomed guest.

Jim picked up the phone.
"Staff Sgt. Stewart" he answered formally.
"Hi Jim," I said. "Fancy playing surrogate daddy?"
There followed a worrying silence. Finally he said, "You mean you want me to meet your children – I can meet your children?"
"No, I want to sell your sperm," I replied sardonically.
He burst out laughing.
"Mine wouldn't be any good, I've had the snip, I fire blanks," he informed me.
Mental note: – If and when *it* happens, I won't have to go back on the pill!
"Babs, you know I would love to meet your children but I thought they were with their father?"
I glanced out of the window again, the children were now sitting on their cases and David had his arm around Lou.
"He hasn't turned up Jim. They've been waiting over an hour now."
"I'm off this afternoon, what's your plan?" he asked.
I told him my plan was to get a picnic together and take them to Castle Park in Colchester. He could show up anytime after 2 pm.
"Forget the picnic Babs, give them something now and I will feed all of you later," he said. I accepted and replaced the phone onto the receiver. Lovely man, I decided.

I banged on the window, beckoning to the children. Reluctantly, they picked up their cases and walked slowly back into the house.

"Should we play the daddy game?" asked Lou, hugging my leg, looking up at me with eyes that could break your heart.

"No sweetie," I said, hugging her, "WE are going to Castle Park and WE are going to have such fun."

"What if he turns up and we aren't here," asked a tearful David.

"He won't," I snapped back, immediately regretting it as his tears started to flow freely.

"Group hug," I said, opening my arms to him. Reluctantly he came over to me and I knelt on the floor and gathered my children into my arms. I felt so guilty because part of me was glad he hadn't arrived. I hated them going away with their father, remembering Lou telling me, "He smells and he smokes funny smelling cigarettes and gets silly."

It hadn't taken me long to work out that he was smoking cannabis as well as drinking.

Concerned, I had phoned Jasmine, my solicitor, for advice.

"Very little can be done," she had told me. "There has to be proof and even then, judges today are so keen to involve fathers in their children's lives, they would probably still allow supervised meetings. Do you really want that? Do you want Social Workers in yours and their lives? Anyway, from what you tell me about him, he will probably lose interest soon – it's *you* he wants to control."

I knew she was right and yes, he was showing signs of losing interest in his children. There was hope yet, I thought guiltily.

The journey to Colchester was in sombre silence, although Louise slept most of the way. David sat grim faced not even pretending to drive, I actually missed the roaring of his imaginary car engine.
We parked the car and went toward the swings, Lou running happily ahead. I was always amazed at how she appeared to shrug off 'bad things'.
"Go play with Lou David," I said, gently steering my son toward the swings. He reluctantly left my side and went to play with his sister although she was almost impossible to keep up with.
I looked around the park and spotted Jim walking determinedly toward me, broad grin on his face, occasionally scanning the playing children, probably trying to recognise which two belonged to me. I had described them to him – David, with his bright red hair standing up in an outgrowing crew cut and the effervescent Lou, who would probably be organising a group of children to do this and do that and sure enough, she was.

Jim sat next to me on the blanket, giving me a tiny kiss on my cheek.
"That one," he said pointing at David, as ever on the periphery of the on going fun. "And that one," he laughed, pointing to Lou who was busy trying to organise some complicated game, the rules of which existed only in her own head.

David was watching her from a distance. He glanced over at me and, spotting the powerful man at my side, sprinted towards us, never taking his suspicious eyes off Jim. Panting, he squeezed his tiny body between us.

"Hello young man, my name's Jim Stewart, I'm a friend of your mother's." Jim put out a large, immaculately clean hand to David, who placed his tiny one in the palm, unable to return the grip but getting it gently shaken.

Lou, spotting a change in the family demographics, came charging over, nearly knocking me over as she hurled herself at me then planted herself in my lap, tiny arms around my neck in a vice like grip.

She didn't look at Jim until he gently touched her shoulder and said,

"Hello, you must be Louise."

She wiggled around to face him, covering her eyes with open fingers, feigning shyness, for this was certainly not part of my little girl's make up.

"Lou," she corrected him – 'awkward little thing', I thought, if he had said Lou, she would have insisted on Louise.

"I thought you might like to come back to camp with me," Jim invited, "join me for some dinner."

"Camp?" asked David and I assumed he was thinking of tents and bonfires. My children were not aware that Colchester was a garrison town. Soldiers clad in different uniforms no longer walked the streets or packed the pubs and restaurants – well those they were allowed into. With all the trouble in Northern Ireland and the constant attacks on the military, they were now forced to wear civilian clothes in town, however, with their cropped hair and always slightly behind the time fashion, they somehow still stood out.

"I'm in the army," Jim told David, who immediately showed interest, being fascinated in all things which he thought part of the male domain.

"Where's your gun then?" asked Lou, moving from my lap to Jims, deciding now that this man was to be trusted. She opened his smart navy blue blazer expecting to find a gun in a holster, cowboy style.

"It's locked away," he laughed, not attempting to stop her search but instead turning his pockets out for her to survey.

We followed Jim's car back to camp – the children wide-eyed when, at the gates, our car was pulled over and searched – underneath, in the boot, under the bonnet – and when the good humoured soldiers searched inside, they joked with the children about smuggling sweets into camp.

That done, we drove further, David staring in wonder at all the different army vehicles, many of them in desert camouflage having recently returned from 'Operation Desert Storm' – the military initiative taking place at that time in the middle-east – which had been caused by a dispute over oil. Iraq had annexed Kuwait and in January 1991 the United States, supported by allied forces including the UK, began Kuwait's liberation.

Jim was not happy at being left behind to run the officers' mess whilst many of his comrades were away fighting. However, selfishly, I felt I needed him more.

The meal in the Sergeants' Mess was a feast and the few there dining with us made a real fuss of the children who were lapping up the attention.

Following the meal, Louise dozing contented on my lap, I watched Jim and the others as they tried to teach David to salute and march. With a blue UN cap perched on his head, he concentrated hard and although he mastered the salute, his uncoordinated little body refused to master the march. He struggled on but his right leg went with his right arm and his left leg with his left arm as he attempted to keep in step with the big burly soldiers. I was afraid, at times, he would be trampled.

"Time to go home," I called, noting the disappointment, for very different reasons, on both Jim and David's face.

Jim carried the now sleepy David and I carried Lou back to my car. I watched as he gently strapped the children into their seats.

"Can I see you all tomorrow?"

I smiled at the *all*.

"We could go to that place you love so much, Mersea is it? I'll get the chef to prepare a picnic to beat all picnics, please say yes Babs, I have so enjoyed today, your kids are wonderful – that little David was trying so hard ..."

Before he could finish I laughed and said "yes, YES ... we would love to see you tomorrow."

101

Checking the children were indeed asleep and that no other inquisitive eyes were watching him, he gave me a long passionate kiss. I was the first to pull away, breathless. He gave me a knowing smile and said,

"Drive carefully, I'll see you tomorrow."

On the way home, there was once again silence in the car. I was lost in my thoughts and the children were fast asleep, the daddy and the pain he had caused that day, at least for now, forgotten.

The sun shone down on Mersea Island, in the distance I could see Jim building sandcastles with the children, most of the time with Lou sprawled across his back, arms around his neck, as he knelt there.

I lay back, eyes closed, content and happy for the first time in months.

I remembered reluctantly, when we had arrived home the previous evening, David had dashed indoors to play the answer phone.

"Nothing," he looked at me, the disappointment showing on his face.

I knew he had expected a message from Bob.

"Doesn't matter," said Lou walking in, rubbing her eyes sleepily, cuddling a grubby teddy bear, the one I was plotting to get away from her and stick in the washing machine,

"Jim can be the daddy now," she added intuitively, as no names had been mentioned. She then took herself to the stairs and almost crawled up, she was so tired.

There is nothing better in my eyes, than a child choosing to go to bed because it is exhausted from fun and play.

I let her go and turned to David, sitting him next to me on the sofa, wishing I could take the pain away.

Although I wanted to rant and rave and tell him what a selfish, useless, thoughtless, bastard his father was, I felt, as usual, that I must protect my child by finding excuses for his errant father's behaviour. "Something really urgent probably came up," I finally said, fingers crossed behind my back.

"Did you have a nice time today?" I asked, desperate to steer away from the present topic.

David suddenly rewarded me with a beaming grin.

"It was great," he said. "Did you see me marching with the soldiers?... Wasn't the food great? ... Did you see all those lorries? ... Want to watch me salute?" With that he had leapt to his feet and started marching around the room in the now familiar, uncoordinated way, then stopping in front of me, he gave me a smart salute, all thoughts of his father gone.

'You lose again Bob', I thought, slyly.

Jim threw himself next to me on the blanket and planted a massive kiss on my lips. I pushed him away, worried the children would see and they did. Were they worried? Not a bit of it. They stood there grinning and making silly noises. David tried to whistle but failing miserably, inadvertently created another game, as Jim spent the next half hour trying to teach them both the skill. I laughed at their little freckled faces, huge cheeks blown out in the effort, lips pursed and nothing but air coming out.

"Well you do it," Jim invited and as I tried, he immediately planted a kiss on my pursed lips causing more hilarity from the children.

"Let's eat," I said quickly, unused to such displays of affection, especially in front of David and Lou.

I opened the large cooler bag and we tucked into what was indeed a superb picnic, carefully prepared for us by the officers' mess Chef. There were chicken legs and wings, cocktail sausages, tiny sandwiches with every filling possible. There were prawns, neatly wrapped in thinly sliced ham, a selection of cheeses, fruit and biscuits and tiny little cakes and sweets with the names, David and Louise carefully piped in icing on the top of each and every one.

There was a cool bottle of superb white wine for Jim and me and several different small bottles of pure fruit juice for the children. Their eyes were agog as they stared at all the food. I barely had enough money to provide a staple diet let alone all these treats. I allowed them to eat what they liked, in whatever order they chose, until inevitably the box stood with only the melting ice packs and a couple of bottles of juice inside it.

Full of food, unable to move very far, the children selected shells from around the edge of the blanket. I still have those shells today, displayed in a basket on the edge of my bath, in memory of that glorious day – the day that marked the true beginning of my wonderful return to a life of normality.

My relationship with Jim went from strength to strength. I was eventually able to tell him about the terrible day Bob had attacked me, injuring me so badly, mentally and physically. I told him about running away with the children, about the kindly couple at the hotel in Colchester. I painfully recalled returning home and finding the house in such a terrible mess. I even told him of my web of safety, my shameful drinking and the nightmare of the divorce.

That night, he took me to bed and made love to me for the first time. It was truly wonderful. He awoke in me feelings that had lain dormant for so many years. He made love to me for hours exploring every inch of my still, painfully thin body and the miracle was, when he lay back exhausted, I was able to make love to him.

We slept in each other's arms until the sun shone through my bedroom curtains and I shook him awake in panic.

"The children," I said. "You have to go. They can't find us like this."

No sooner had the words left my lips when the door was pushed open and there stood David and Louise, carrying tea and toast, smiling from ear to ear, as if finding us together in bed was the most natural thing on earth. Jim feigned sleep as I hustled them out of the room. When we heard their steps running down the stairs again we looked at each other in total amazement, then holding each other fell back onto the pillows in hysterics.

Later that year, Jim took the next step of inviting us all to his home town of Bolton to meet his family and most importantly his two teenage daughters, Kirsty 14 and Kerry just turned 13. "Not my choice of names," he had pointed out.
I was concerned for all of us, although I had mentally tried to prepare myself for this day.
I had felt a strange jealousy every time he drove the 200 miles home to see his girls. Used to him being away on exercise for weeks on end, the children never questioned these absences but I knew they saw Jim as being theirs and I was worried how they would feel and indeed how I would feel, sharing his affection.

The journey to Lancashire was wonderful. We had to stop on several occasions to let the children stretch their legs, as they had never travelled so far in a car before.
The changing scenery and indeed the changing weather, captivated me, the clear roads of the south replaced with bright white snow covering the roads and the moors of the north. The children sat peering out of the car windows in wide-eyed wonder. This was the first time they had been out of Essex.

Jim's mother, an elderly crippled widow, had a cold unwelcoming home. She had a large, bad tempered dog that growled and eyed us suspiciously, as indeed, did she – well she didn't growl but I am sure she would have liked to. Jim was obviously the apple of her eye and she fussed around him, asking if he was hungry and blatantly exclaiming it must have been tiring having two such young children in *his* car.

David and Louise clung to me nervously, frightened of this woman who ignored them and a dog that looked at them as if they were its next meal.

No beds had been prepared and Jim left us with his mother as he rushed upstairs to do something about it.

That night the children and I shared a cold uncomfortable bed, cuddling each other for warmth. Louise announced she wanted to go home, David however, remained quiet. Jim slept in what had been his bedroom 20 years ago, still decorated as if he were a teenage boy.

The next morning I was horrified to be told by his mother – whom I swear found a spiteful pleasure in it – that Jim had gone to see his daughters. We were left trapped with her and the dog with no idea when Jim would return. Her eyes were pinned to the television and it wasn't until Lou said she was hungry, that she broke the silence and unwillingly offered to make the children a sandwich. Not used to being unable to make conversation, I finally gave up, wrapped the children up warmly and together we went in search of food. It had been very dark when we arrived and I was dismayed to find ourselves surrounded by houses, not a shop in sight. I had no intention of returning to the inhospitable house or the unfriendly woman and her dog, so the children and I walked and walked and eventually got completely lost. It was getting dark and Lou was tired complaining she was hungry and her feet were sore. As usual, David didn't complain but hung on to me as we sat on a bench, resting our aching feet and listening to our tummies rumbling.

'If only I could remember the address or had had the foresight to make a note of the telephone number' I thought to myself. We sat there shivering for what seemed like an hour.

A car drew up beside us and Jim's annoyed face peered out of the window.

"What do you think you are playing at?" he asked, as the children scrambled into the warmth of the car.

I sat next to him in the passenger seat. "We were hungry," I said calmly.

"Mum's cooked dinner, we were worried," he barked at me.

I smiled sweetly at him and asked him to join me outside. I got out of the car and to his surprise, sat back down on the bench he had just found us sitting on.

When he joined me, still smiling and keeping my voice low, I said,

"Don't you ever speak to me like that again! *You* left us alone, I had no idea when you would return, we were not offered anything to eat until around 11 o'clock when Lou complained of being hungry and then it was with some reluctance. So here we are in the middle of Beirut and you say *you* were worried!"

"We've found sweets," called David from the back of the car, "Can we have them?"

"No," Jim shouted back. "They are for my girls!"

He realised that he had made a very big mistake when he looked at my face and saw the fury in my eyes. I said, very calmly, the chill in my voice matching the chill of the weather,

"Well here is what we will do. We will go back to your mother's, I will pack our bags and if you would be so kind as to lend me some money and drive us to the station, I will take the children home by train – tonight."

Jim went to say something but I got up, went to the car and climbed in. As he joined me I turned to the children and with a smile on my face said,

"Of course you can have the sweets, Jim was teasing you."

The drive was silent, the children blissfully unaware of the unfamiliar atmosphere as they munched away on Kirsty and Kerry's sweets. I noted we were only five minutes away from his mother's house.

I told the children to sit and wait in the lounge as I marched upstairs to pack our bags and before very long Jim joined me.

"They are scoffing down shepherd's pie," he laughed. I didn't turn around but continued throwing things into two cases.

"Please don't go," he begged, "I'm sorry, so very sorry, I didn't think."

109

I spun round, feeling free to lose my temper,

"I, we, have had far too many years of a bloody man not bloody thinking," I said, trying not to shout. I didn't want the children to hear me.

"I know, I know, I know," he said striding toward me, horrified when I backed off, my hands held up in front of me as if to fend off an attack.

"Oh my God Babs don't! I would never hurt you – surely you know that?"

I sat weakly down on the edge of the bed, panic and anger and hunger all mixed in together. He sat with me and I didn't fight him when he took me in his arms.

I have no excuse," he said, "Except to say my girls got very upset when I told them about you and the children. I didn't feel I could leave them like that."

"They are teenagers," I replied, quietly fighting back the moment's panic I had felt.

"It doesn't make it any easier," he argued gently. "I love them as much as you love your two and I don't get to see them as often. I spend more time with your children and well Kirsty and Kerry, they worked that out and were hurt. Please stay, I so want you to meet them."

I was overwhelmed with a feeling of foreboding as I looked at his handsome face and his troubled eyes but all I could think of saying was,

"There's truble at' mill."

"Aye," he replied in his broad Lancashire accent, "And me best pigeon's not cum back."

We both laughed and I agreed to give it a couple more days, especially as he promised we wouldn't be spending long with his daughters and he would show us the moors and Bolton.

"They are having their nails done in the afternoon, so we only have a couple of hours in the morning, they are being dropped off here by their mother," he told me.

As we walked back downstairs together, I felt apprehension return and his words, 'they are having their nails done' went over and over in my mind.

KERRY AND KIRSTY

They sat sullenly on the tatty sofa and, to my nasty spiteful delight, I noticed Jim's mother was just as cool with Jim's daughters, Kirsty and Kerry, as she was with my children and me.

David and Louise were content having earlier consumed a large breakfast, cooked, however, by Jim. He was a very talented chef, which suited me as I hated cooking and had a habit of setting fire to things, kitchens included. His mother had fussed around him until he had said,

"Go away mother, I can cope, I do all the cooking at Barbara's."

She glared at me and I gave her my best 'Yeah, got something to say?' look and went back to trying to make small talk with the two visitors.

"Look," said Lou, going over innocently to Kerry, taking with her a large sketchpad. Realising the children had nothing to play with Jim had rushed out that morning and bought them both a sketchpad and crayons.

"I've drawn you," she continued, pushing the pad underneath Kerry's nose. To my amazement, Kerry leant forward and picked up my little girl. Smiling, she stroked her long, black unruly hair and pushed her fringe away from her eyes.

"Oh that's lovely," she said, giving her a little squeeze. I started to warm to this awkward teenager and smiled at her and was immediately rewarded with an equally friendly smile.

David looked as if he was going to move toward Kirsty, thought better of it and went back to his work of art, which may or may not have been an army lorry. She ignored us all, preferring to examine her beautifully manicured fingernails. 'Hmmm I thought, they don't look as if they need *doing*.'

She smiled warmly at her father when he entered the room carrying soft drinks and biscuits and I noticed, with interest, that he chose to sit on the arm of the sofa next to Kirsty, rather than in-between his two daughters.

This was not missed by his eldest daughter who, glancing over, gave a little shrug of acceptance and carried on talking to Lou about her work of art, making suggestions as to what colours she could use to enhance it.

Kirsty and Jim joked and whispered to each other until he caught my angry stare.

He leapt to his feet,

"Lunch," he said. "Where does everyone want to go?"

"McDonalds," Kerry, David and Lou said in unison.

"KFC," said Kirsty.

So off we went to Kentucky Fried Chicken, Kirsty sitting in the front of the car, next to her father. She had rushed out of the house, climbed into the car and stared out of the window at me challengingly. I opened the car door and stooping down, smiled at her and said,

"Why don't you sit next to your father?" then closed the door again with more than necessary force and climbed into the back with Kerry and my two children.

"Why is she sitting there?" said Lou, giving Kirsty a little poke in the back.

"Ouch!" squealed Kirsty, as if she had been stabbed. She looked imploringly at her father who turned around and glared at Louise. She, in turn, stuck her thumb in her mouth, leaned her head against Kerry's shoulder as she strapped her into her seat and stared innocently back at him.

'Oh dear' I thought. 'This is not going well.'

Four of us chatted away whilst eating our meal. Kirsty said nothing. Occasionally Jim asked his youngest if she was OK or how was her meal, whilst I planned *not* to do the Heimlich manoeuvre should she start to choke on a chicken bone. 'Bitchy Babs, very bitchy,' I grinned to myself.

Kerry and I were now getting on like a house on fire and she was excellent with the children, cutting their food into small pieces and gently wiping their caked in tomato sauce mouths with a serviette.

Our plates empty she turned to me and said,

"Come and see this dress I'm going to buy later."

Throwing a 'stay put' look at David and Louise, I left the restaurant with Kerry and arm in arm we walked to a nearby dress shop.

She pointed out an amazingly short red, Lycra dress, with long sleeves, which I imagined would hug her slightly overweight body, showing every lump, every bulge.

"Is that the only colour it comes in?" I asked cautiously.

"No," she replied, staring in pleasure at the horribly expensive dress displayed on the perfect body of a shop window mannequin.

"It comes in black too. Do you think that would be better?"

"Oh yes," I replied hastily. "And buy a size larger than you usually wear, then you won't constantly be pulling it down at the hem to cover your embarrassment," I advised.

"Good idea batman," she laughed, good-naturedly.

We walked back to the restaurant to find Jim and Kirsty chatting away merrily whilst my two sat bored, kicking their heels, obviously not included in the conversation going on in front of them.

In fact, I noted, Jim had paid my children no attention at all, apart from his unwarranted glare at Lou, since the arrival of Kerry and Kirsty.

I pushed the thought to the back of my mind as Jim, looking at his watch, told his girls they had better go or they would be late for their nail appointment.

"Can I have mine done too?" asked Lou, looking at the tiny nails on her left hand.

"No!" snapped Kirsty.

"Yours don't need doing," said David, putting a protective arm around his little sister and throwing an angry look at Kirsty that belied his years.

Kirsty threw her arms around her father and kissed him, holding onto him tightly, Kerry then gave him a hug then turned to me and hugged me too. As Kirsty strode out of the restaurant, Kerry cuddled and kissed both of my children, promising to see them again soon, and followed her taller, slimmer, younger sister. She alone turned back and waved, as they both disappeared into the crowd of Bolton shoppers.

I was very relieved as we walked around Bolton's busy town centre – Jim a couple of paces in front of us – that he hadn't as yet, asked me what I thought of his two daughters. Although I could have sung the praises of Kerry, I would have struggled to say a decent word about his youngest and, now obvious to me, favourite daughter. I could honestly say I loved my two equally and couldn't understand how a parent could play favourites with their children. Having seen many family photos displayed on Jim's mothers old Welsh dresser, I noted that Kerry was more like the Stewart family. Plainer than her sister, she was a tall, stocky girl, with neat, short dark hair and round features and she had her father's warm brown eyes. Kirsty was still taller and much slimmer, with long curly auburn hair – a shade darker than David's bright red hair – that framed her pretty face but, unlike my son's warm, sparkling eyes, hers of the same colour, were cold.

Jim suddenly seemed to remember we were with him and turned around and reached his arms out to my children who, for the first time, took his hands a little reluctantly, looking back at me for unspoken approval.
We later drove out to the beautiful countryside and I looked in wonder at the tiny funnels protruding

from the earth. Jim explained that they were the breathing funnels for the miles of mine shafts, hundreds of feet below. We stopped on the moors to allow the children to run and play and the atmosphere between us relaxed.

"They are not like your two," Jim said, looking at David and Louise, as they chased each other, rosy cheeked, coats flying open, oblivious of the cold weather.

"Yours are little extroverts," he explained. "Mine are both very shy."

"Kerry's adorable," I said to him pointedly.

He looked at me quizzically.

"And Kirsty?" he asked.

"Rude and unkind," I replied, refusing to lie.

He stepped away, looking at me with angry eyes. I held his gaze, fighting back the anger I felt rising in mine.

"She just doesn't know you," he said.

"Mine were never rude to you Jim, never, not once, not even when they first met you and yes, Kerry was indeed at first shy, but at least she tried and I really liked her."

"Kirsty however, was petulant, rude and unkind. She treated David and Louise with total disregard and they are so little and innocent and wanted to be friends."

With that I stomped back to the car, shouting sarcastically,

"I assume it's OK for me to sit in the front?"

With that I sat down and *gently* closed the car door, furious with Kirsty, furious with Jim, furious with myself, furious with an unfair world that continued to throw hurdles to leap over in front of me.

For 10 minutes I watched him play with the children, occasionally furtively glancing back at me whilst I sat stony faced in the car.

An enormous sadness threatened to overwhelm me as I realised that this man, with whom I'd been slowly falling in love, would never love my children as much as he loved his own, they would always take second place and that would never do.

I sat there in silence, slowly building an impenetrable wall around my heart and there it would stay, for many years, until I felt my children were safe from my mistakes.

We met the girls on one more occasion that trip. Kerry was her warm friendly self, sweeping the children up into her arms and planting kisses on their smiling faces – Kirsty stood aloof, gripping her father's arm who, to his credit, forced her this time into conversation with me.

More surprisingly perhaps, Jim's mother decided she liked my children and me.

"You make him so happy," she had revealed to me in her kitchen one morning.

Earlier we had almost had an argument when she virtually accused me of being lazy, as I never prepared our meals. Never one to back off from a fight I had asked her,

"If you were cooking and someone was constantly looking over your shoulder asking why you were adding some ingredient or the other and why you weren't adding another, what would you say?"

"I would say 'do it your bloody self,'" she retorted, then smiled at me, instantly getting the point. I winked at her. "Exactly," I said.

This really broke the ice. We sat in the kitchen, the only really warm room in the house with its ever hot, wood burning cooking range, chatting away like old friends until she started to show me old photos from a pile of albums.

I was in for another shock.

"That's Jim's first wife," she said, tapping an arthritic finger on an old yellowing photograph showing a very young Jim with a dark-haired beauty, obviously, from their dress, a wedding picture. "And these two, they are his son and daughter. His wife went off with one of his friends, broke his heart," his mother went on.

I couldn't speak. I had no idea Jim had been married twice, let alone have another two children, who must, by now, be in their early twenties. Luckily, Jim's mother went to put the kettle on the hob, not noticing my look of horror.

"Does he see them often?" I asked, peering intently at the two little faces smiling at me from the photograph.

"Never," came the shocking reply. "It's like they don't exist, not since the other two were born."

So Jim had four children but only had enough love for two. How desperately sad, I thought, and how could I ever expect him to love mine if he couldn't love his own?

I tucked all this knowledge away whilst we lunched at McDonalds, much to princess Kirsty's disgust, refusing to eat anything. Instead, she hugged a strawberry milk shake, which I swear was gradually curdling in her grip as she chatted away about her wonderful mother.

"We love her going away for the whole night," she enthused, wincing slightly as her sister, sitting opposite, landed a kick on her shin. This didn't faze her as she blundered on.

"She leaves us a few bottles of wine and sweets and cakes!"

I nearly choked on my food, 'out of the mouths of babes' I thought.

Jim's back straightened visibly. He smiled at his youngest daughter and asked nonchalantly, "How many bottles darling?"

"Oh just a couple each," she said, smiling at me, as if she had scored precious points.

Kerry sighed in defeat, "Dad, we don't drink it all," she claimed.

"We sooooooo do," Kirsty argued. "You were sick last time," she laughed.

Kerry leant back in defeat and stole a look at me. I tried to smile at her reassuringly but knew I couldn't hide my natural concern from her.

Turning to me Jim said,

"OK if I drop you back at mums? Think I'll pop in and have a word with their mother."

"Someone should," was my reply.

Much later Jim arrived back at his mother's house, worry and anger etched on his face. He asked her to take the children into the kitchen and sat down with me, his head in his hands.

"She told me to *butt out*," he said. "Can you believe that, *butt out*? I won't be able to take a commission, I'll have to move back here when I retire, keep an eye on things. I'm always too far away."

"That's in three years," I said, "that's too late."

"What can I do?" he asked me desperately.

"Social Services, at least threaten her with that," I suggested.

He went into the hall to phone his errant wife. I heard him getting angry but when he came back into the room he looked slightly happier.

"It worked," he said relieved. "Alcohol is now off the menu."

That night in bed, holding onto my own two children, I took comfort in knowing they were loved by me and safe with me. Jim had always claimed his former wife was a wonderful mother. Now he knew differently he was going to have to spend less time with me and mine and more time with his own family. Remembering his other two children I mentally added, with sadness in my heart, another layer of bricks to my wall.

Our relationship lasted another three years and most of it was good. He was very kind to the children, often buying them those things they would never have had without him around. He bought their first bikes for example – they weren't brand new but after he had expertly repaired them and painted them, adding bells and pumps and little bags on the back, they might just as well have been.

He often told me he loved me and I really believe he did but once up, I couldn't tear down the wall around my heart.

I had started an Access course at Braintree College and when I had important exams, Jim took the children to Bolton with him to give me time to study. Now aged 11 and 8, they were sad little souls when they returned home. David quietly told me one day that Jim's daughters had wanted him to stay the weekend with them, as their mother was away – which he did, leaving them alone for two long days with his mother – who no longer left the house – and a dog that growled and barked every time they moved.

"Louise was so upset mum," David had said, failing to hide his own disappointment. "He was gone for ages and didn't phone or anything."

Gradually I teased more and more information from my children and discovered that, although showing them love and affection in my presence, away from me Jim was often cool and aloof and never defended them in times of strife with his mother or with his daughter Kirsty.

That was it really. This relationship had to end, my children were far more important than any relationship of mine. So I met Jim one more time and told him it was over. I told him that the children and I were a package deal – 'love me love my kids.'

"No one is going to love your children as much as they love their own," he had argued desperately. "And I do my best." But I remembered his first two children – he was certainly failing to *do his best* with them.

"I know," I said gently. "So I intend staying on my own until they are independent. I'll become mother Teresa if necessary but I will not have my children hurt again by any relationship of mine."

And so we parted. He tried for months, phoning me, inviting me to functions at camp, even tempting me through my children to various children's activities like a huge bonfire night, Christmas parties and trips to the seaside, but I stayed resolute. I took on a life of celibacy, for 10 long years, and did I miss having a man in my life? Not one bit!!

KEELE

As I walked across Keele University's beautiful campus in Staffordshire, feeling the autumn chill in the air on this bright October morning, I expected someone to tap me on the shoulder and ask me what the hell I thought I was doing there. Wasn't I Barbara Cunningham, mother of two from Essex, who'd failed her GCE exams in 1996?

I was totally lost, I had been trying to find the Criminology and the Psychology departments for what seemed like hours.

I was overwhelmed by the size of the place – Braintree College would have fitted comfortably into the Library alone.

I stood by the church staring down the slope at the mass of students and academics milling about. This was fresher week, what was it going to be like when the hundreds of other students arrived?

"You look as lost as I am," said a friendly voice and I turned to see the pretty face of a young girl who must have been in her early 20's. "I'm Beverly," she said, leaning her hands on her knees, her long blonde hair falling over her face. "My feet are killing me, I've transferred from Middlesborough, hated it there. Don't you just love this campus?"

"I would if I could find the Criminology and Psychology departments," I said wearily.

"Wow me too," she laughed. "They are my principals and I'm doing Biology and Sociology as subsids."

"Wow back at ya," I grinned. "They are my subsids too, so we could be seeing a lot of each other."

Beverly and I then went on a journey of discovery, picking up other lost and nervous freshers on our way. We were aged from between 19 and 60, from all different races and creeds.

'I am going to love this,' I thought to myself and I still wasn't absolutely sure how, at this point in my life, I had arrived here.

"What are you all filling in?" I had asked one morning, walking into the refectory and joining the other mature students who were with me on the access course at Braintree College. They were bent over, busily filling in complicated looking forms and comparing notes.

"Our UCAS forms," said Tim looking up.

"What are UCAS forms?" I asked him.

"Babs, what the hell have you been doing here for the last 3 months?" he laughed.

"Errm the Access Course?" I replied, returning his smile but still puzzled.

"Access to what?" he asked.

"I know this one," I grinned. "Access to a qualification to help me get a job and crawl out of the poverty trap", I replied.

Several of the others now looked up and exchanged exaggerated glances of disbelief. Tim and I were known as the group clowns and they were waiting for us to go into some hastily prepared routine.

"Now sit down and try to concentrate," said Tim. He was only 27, tall, dark and handsome and I adored him. He was intelligent and funny and hard working and we had clicked immediately, proving, once again, that age has nothing to do with friendship.

"The course you have been on for the past three months has beeeeeeeeen … wait for it … drum roll please … access to Higher Education … applause!!"

"What's that then ay?" I asked in my best Essex accent.

"Oh my God Babs," Tim feigned despair – or was it real despair – as he put his head in his hands?

"I thought this course *was* Higher Education," I was now very confused.

Desperate to get away from the boredom of everyday life and having been promised a job with Jen and Lou at their nursery school, I had sat the entrance exam for the NNEB course (National Nursery Examination Board) at Braintree College. Within a week of the exam I received a phone call asking me to attend the college and meet Mrs Godfrey, the student adviser. It was 1993 and as I hadn't sat an exam since the 1960's, when I had failed all but two of my GCE's, I feared the worst. I assumed I had failed the NNEB exam and was going to be offered a re-sit.

I looked at Louise playing happily on the kitchen floor and hoped Mrs Godfrey didn't have a floor-standing potted plant.

Mrs Godfrey was a pleasant, slightly built woman, who looked at least 10 years my junior.

I threw a worried glance at Louise who had already started to wriggle on the seat I had placed her on with a warning 'STAY' look in my eyes. She sat back resolutely and I turned back to Mrs Godfrey who was studying what looked to be my exam papers.

'Oh Lord,' I thought, 'wasn't life hard enough without putting myself through this?'

"Brilliant," said Mrs Godfrey smiling at me. "You scored 100%! Absolutely brilliant."

To say I was 'gob smacked' would be a massive understatement – I had never been praised for an exam result in my life before! As I sat there with my mouth open, she continued,

"Our concern is that the NNEB course will fail to stretch your educational capabilities and we will lose you as a student."

I wasn't really listening as she went on about 'access courses' and 'only a year of my time', I could only think … '100%!'

I came out of my stupor when I heard her say "next week."

"I beg your pardon," I asked, slightly embarrassed at my loss of concentration for one so brilliant!

"We are holding a week's intensive entrance course next week. It's usually a month, but you have missed that one, however we are sure you can cope. At the end a decision will be made as to whether or not you qualify for the Access Course which starts at the end of September. Are you interested?"

Not really understanding what she was talking about, having been lost in my own thoughts for at least half of the conversation, I happily agreed. T's crossed and all the dots put in the right places, I signed several different forms and Mrs Godfrey, shaking my hand, bade me farewell and said she looked forward to seeing me at 9.30 sharp on Monday morning.

"So what is an Access Course?" Kate later asked, having promised to look after Louise the following week.
"I have no idea," I laughed. "I think it's just a qualification to get us oldies back into work and off benefits."
And that's the way it was. The intensive course successfully completed, I started the Access Course the following September, still convinced it was simply a qualification.

So here I was, looking at Tim and the others in bewilderment.
"Oh Lord," said Tim opening his arms to include the others. "We are all here because we want to go to university and get degrees having for some reason or the other never taken 'A' levels."
"I can't go to university," I said, now quite shocked. "I've got kids and I'm not clever enough."
"I've got six kids", said Kim at the other end of the table, looking depressed.
"That's what this course is all about," said a now very frustrated Tim, "To prepare us for university,

to show that we *are* good enough. Fill in the dam form and shut up," he laughed, pushing a blank UCAS form at me.

'Oh well,' I thought. 'May as well fill it in, no university is going to want me anyway'!!!

Amazingly, they did! I had been offered places at three universities – Keele the only one to ask to see essays from college for Psychology – and I had to attend an interview before being accepted to study Criminology.

'A method in their madness', I had wryly thought, as I drove onto the beautiful campus on a hot July day. Anyone seeing this lovely university would have no trouble visualising living here happily for the next three years.

Always slow to pick up information, it was only then that I had realised Keele was a dual honours degree university. That meant I had to study two principal subjects and another two subsidiary subjects, these two had to be completed in the first year. What on earth had I taken on?

It was hard – it was very, very hard. I was 200 hundred miles away from my friends, I had two children to look after, money as usual was tight, so I was cleaning a pub before going to lectures and doing bar work and waiting on tables at the weekends and during vacations. And there was so much work for my degree, endless lectures, essays and lab reports and preparation for group work and presentations. If I had an evening free, the children and I would go to the university library. I would find the books I needed and they would photocopy the chapters I selected.

Studying for exams was the worst. They came straight after school holidays, so I had to revise during school holidays. David had just turned 13 and Louise was now 10. They had reached that dreadful 'fight over everything' stage. I still had to shop and prepare meals and break up fights, not really convivial with studying for a dual honours degree and no excuse for missed deadlines or poor work.
Then, just after Christmas, during my second year, our little world received another blow.

I had rented a lovely bungalow in a tiny, pretty village called Madeley, complete with a duck pond, although this was referred to as *the pool* as streams flowed in and out of it. Madeley was only 15 minutes from the university and the small town of Newcastle Under Lyme was only 20 minutes away. Driving to the village, in the distance we could see the Welsh mountains and from our lounge patio doors, green hills, trees and fields. It was a complete contrast to the noisy main road we had lived on in Braintree. Here it was quiet and tranquil. On a clear night you could see millions of bright stars in the sky and in March 1997 we were able to stare in wonder at the Hale-Bopp Comet as it hovered above us, its bright tail streaming out behind.

The bungalow was fully furnished, so we had taken only a few precious things with us – the stereo my brother had given us, my lovely antique dressing table – a present from my parents – pictures and photographs and of course the children's games and toys and our books.

David and Louise were both in walking distance of their schools and the village had everything you could possibly want, doctors and dentists, a tiny supermarket, an excellent butchers, a small haberdashery that also sold the children's school uniforms, a post office and of course a village church and a local pub. It also had an excellent Indian Restaurant, a superb Chinese Takeaway and the best fish and chip shop on earth.

The children were naturally nervous to find themselves in such a different environment. The local people had an unfamiliar accent and we needed to learn and understand colloquialisms. For example if you were ill, you were *laid up*, a hill was a *bank*, the snow didn't settle it would *stick* and unlike the *love* and *darlin'* of the South, here in the Midlands, you were called *duck*.

I was very content in Madeley and the children soon settled down at their new schools and made friends.

I had intended returning to Braintree at least once a month to check on things but due to my uni work load and my jobs, it was 18 months before I returned. It had been a particularly harsh winter and I was horrified when I entered the house to find the pipes had burst and the kitchen was flooded.

I sought the help of Jeff, a man to whom I'd sold furniture when I had been desperate for money. He had befriended the children and me and when I told him I was moving to the Midlands, he had offered to store my furniture.

Within an hour he met me at the house and assured me that most of our belongings were salvable. There and then I decided it was time to say goodbye to the house where I had lived through so much sadness and struggle. Jeff promised to move everything for me and store it safely in a strong dry warehouse on his land.

"Just leave it to me Babs, take what you need and I will take care of the rest," he had promised.

So, having locked the back door of the house for the last time and giving the key to Jeff, I drove back to Madeley and our little, cosy bungalow.

It came as an enormous blow when, just before Christmas, in my second year at Keele, my landlady announced she had sold the bungalow and we had a month to vacate.

I took time off from uni and went in search of a new home without any luck – it was either too expensive or too horrible to be considered. Eventually, Keele's Student Support department came to my rescue and, after contacting the local council, assured me the children and I were not heading for cardboard city but would be re-housed in Madeley.

Within a few weeks we went to see what was to be our new home. My heart sunk when I saw, for the first time, the shabby old council house we were to live in. The children and I peered through the glass of the filthy windows with rotting wooden frames. We saw old-fashioned open fireplaces in the dining room and lounge. The kitchen was incredibly out of date and a deep puddle covered most of the dirty kitchen floor. The décor was loud and ugly and pictures and brass ornaments were nailed to the walls.

A grey-suited man from the council arrived to show us around the house and things went from bad to worse. The bathroom was quite the most disgusting I had ever seen. The bath was thick with filth, as were the toilets up and downstairs. The heating and water were coal-fired, which meant keeping a fire burning in the lounge if we wanted to be clean and warm. There were only four radiators in the whole house – in two of the three bedrooms, and in the lounge and dining room.

The back garden was enormous, overgrown and surrounded by tall, out of control hedges. There were two ugly and decrepit coalbunkers directly outside the kitchen window and what appeared to be a huge rubbish dump just beyond.

"The council will carry out all necessary repairs and redecorate," the man from the council assured me. "And these properties are due to be updated within the next two years or more."

As we walked back to the bungalow, David took my hand and said,

"It will be alright mummy, you'll see, I'll take care of things, it's going to be our new home, we'll be safe there." And with that he kissed the back of my hand and ran to catch up with Lou who was skipping happily ahead of us. I was once again amazed at the strength of my little people. They were happy as long as we were together, drawing strength from each other.

'Yes,' I decided, 'we *will* be alright, I will make sure we are alright' and as I raced past them I shouted, 'last one home's a sissy.'

"It's all gone," said Jeff.

"What do you mean it's all gone?" I asked puzzled.

"We had a bad storm here a few weeks ago … wind blew the roof off the warehouse … furniture was so badly damaged I had to get rid of it … no insurance … couldn't find your phone number … couldn't let you know."

I sat there stunned, we had only two weeks to go before moving into an unfurnished house and Jeff was telling me I had nothing to put in it, *nothing*!!

"The cooker, the two fridge freezers, what about the washing machine, the children's beds, there must be something?"

"Nothing," he replied, "well you don't have a house to put it in anyway and your place is furnished you said."

"I'm moving Jeff, we have to leave in two weeks, we have a council house a bloody empty council house and you're telling me I have nothing to put in it, I trusted you, you said it would be OK you said ..."

"Not my fault ... nothing signed ... no proof." CLICK the phone went dead.

I rushed into the bathroom and was violently sick into the toilet, I slumped down onto the floor, I couldn't breathe, I was gasping for breath, felt I was going to pass out.

"Mum?" David was standing at the bathroom door.

"Paper bag, quick, mushrooms," I gasped.

David disappeared, I heard him in the kitchen, heard him rummaging around in the fridge and then he reappeared in the bathroom pushing a paper bag with a solitary mushroom in it, toward me. I clamped it to my mouth and started breathing, tried to control my breathing, tried to quell the panic attack that was threatening to overwhelm me.

As I lay slumped on the bathroom floor, David put a cold flannel on my forehead. He was as white as a ghost. Lou appeared in the doorway.

"I'm not picking up all them mushrooms," she said, hands on hips.

"*Those* mushrooms," David and I said in unison, then looked at each other and laughed.

"Why are you both on the floor?" she asked.

David helped me to my feet and helped me into the lounge,

"Mummy isn't well," he said to Louise.

They sat either side of me on the large sofa. My breathing was gradually returning to normal. 'How was I going to tell them, hadn't they been through enough, hadn't I been through enough?'

David was stroking the back of my right hand and assuming that was what one did in an emergency, Lou started to stroke the left.

"It's all gone," I said to them, my voice barely a whisper. "We have nothing, not one stick of furniture."

"I don't understand," David said, shaking his head in bewilderment, "I thought Jeff had it in a shed."

"He said there was a storm, took the roof off the warehouse," I tried to explain.

"Well I for one don't believe him," said Lou shaking her head angrily. "He was always taking our furniture."

"I sold it to him sweetie," I said, putting her hand in mine. But her words made me think. Had he sold it, lied to me?

"I think she's right," said David. "When he came for that old dresser, he was looking in the bookcase, that old one daddy had brought home with the leaded glass in the doors. He said how nice it was and did I think you wanted that to go too? I can remember mummy, I remembered you saying how much you loved it and it was the only decent thing Daddy had come home with and I told him no. He's got it now hasn't he?"

I felt so angry, why had I trusted him? But I knew the answer to that – because he was there when I needed money. This had become confused in my head, it wasn't a kindness, I was selling him furniture and jewellery when I was desperate and probably for half of what it was worth. £20 to me at that time meant a full fridge and full tummies. Or it meant I could buy birthday or Christmas presents, whatever the reason, he had got bargains and now I was pretty sure he had stolen nearly everything I owned.

Leaving the children at home, I walked into the village and sat on a bench by the pool, watching the profusion of wildlife it attracted.

"Babs, you OK duck?"

It was Cheryl, she worked in the local off-licence. She had made me feel very welcome when I had moved to the village. We had bought a bottle of wine from her to have with our dinner of fish and chips, to toast our new life in the village. She had picked up on our southern accents and had told us where the doctor's surgery was and chatted about the schools the children were going to attend. When I felt lonely or just fancied a chat I would walk to the 'offie' and we would sit on crates and drink coffee and she would try to teach me 'Stokie lingo'.

"C'mon," she said, and taking my arm, we walked in silence to the shop.

"Tell me," she said, handing me a box of tissues and a glass of brandy. So I told her the whole sorry story about selling furniture to Jeff and trusting him and the burst pipes and trusting him and leaving the house in Braintree for the last time and trusting him and it was all gone ... everything ... gone.

Neither of us noticed the customer until she approached us and stooped down in front of me and took my hands.

"I'm so sorry," she said, "I couldn't help but hear. I have two single beds and some curtains. I've also got a couple of bookcases and some lamp shades if that would help? I know it's not much," … and her voice trailed away as I started to sob.

After everything I have been through, when I look back, losing all my furniture was one of the most painful events of my life. For a few days the recollection made me dry up. I could find no words to continue writing and this was confusing.

One morning, during the early hours, I chatted online with Lou, in the meantime 21 and at University. She was playing catch up with essays and I was fighting writer's block:

Babs: I had writer's block today for the first time, only wrote a little
Lou: well i wouldn't worry about it, probly just means u need a break
Babs: I'm sure it does I got to the bit about the furniture being stolen, found it upsetting, strange after everything we went through
Lou: theres gonna be lots of stuff you'll find upsetting to bring up, but this'll help you properly move on from it
Babs: dont you think I have?
Lou: i do think you have in the way that matters most, but it takes a very long time to reach a point where you can control how the memories make you feel
Lou: for example writing about the furniture being stolen still upsets you which it will because it

was a huge act of betrayal, but eventually it ought to empower you because of the way you overcame it and found a solution to help you to realise your strength

Lou: all about perspective
Babs: how did you get to be so wise?
Lou: learned from the best baby xxx

As I lay in bed Lou's words, 'the way you overcame it and found a solution,' went over and over in my head.

I recalled one of my father's favourite quotations, which he used to recite when he injured himself doing some DIY job or other about the house. It came from a poem 'Ballad of Sir Andrew Barton', written in the seventeenth century by one of England's famous poets, John Dryden:

" ... I am hurt but I am not slain. I'll lay me down and bleed awhile, and then I'll rise and fight again."

I loved these words when I first heard them as a child, little knowing then how important they would become to me and how often in my life I would adhere to them.

For I did precisely that – I grieved for a few days then pulled myself together again. They were after all just objects, bits of furniture and ornaments, electrical goods. There was of course much, much more than that – he had emptied a four bed roomed family home. I didn't dare itemise what exactly had gone but occasionally things would spring to mind, for example my huge record collection and cassettes and there were gifts from people the children and I loved. Wonderful brass ornaments my brother had lovingly brought back from Saudi. There were other precious items, my children's first pair of shoes, many of their toys, our clothes, bedding, photographs and pictures. The children's first works of art had gone and all our certificates and proof of my qualifications, which would cause so many problems later.

Lou was most upset about her bedroom wardrobe. "All my stickers are on it," she had wailed, whilst David sat grim faced, lost in his own memories of toy cars, ships and aeroplanes, he had patiently and lovingly put together, following complicated instructions and refusing all help.
I swept aside any thoughts of monetary value, these things were priceless, they were gone and I would never have them back, there was no point dwelling on it, I had to start again, and soon.

The first thing I did – something I usually avoided doing – was to phone my sweet sister Jane. I hated having to turn to my family for help, hated having to worry them, but now I had no option.

YOU DON'T KNOW WHAT IT'S LIKE

Jane had lived with her lawyer husband and children for many years in the tax-free utopia of Hong Kong and was now enjoying a 'comfortable life' in England.

I immediately regretted my action, as she was so upset.

"How could he do this too you, Babs, whatever have you done to deserve all this?"

"I'll name them you tick them off," I joked, trying to lighten the conversation as I could hear the worry in her voice.

"You always joke," she said laughing. "I don't know how you cope, I know I couldn't."

And I secretly hoped she would never have to.

"I have some things I don't need," she said. "You are welcome to them, I'll send them to you, have them delivered to your new home on the day you move in. I wasn't sure what I was going to do with it all, don't know why I brought it to the UK from Hong Kong, there must be a God."

'There *must* indeed be a God', I thought, the day we moved into the house, for a huge lorry arrived containing a three peace suite and a coffee table, a double bed, a complete set of rattan bedroom furniture and a wardrobe. There were the most beautiful curtains I had ever seen, enough to cover every window in the house. There was a washing machine that did everything except load the clothes, a dishwasher, (sigh) cutlery and crockery and glasses, some crystal.

I had bought from our landlady, Lou's bed, a picnic table and benches that would be just fine in the kitchen to have our meals on, an ugly teak dresser for storage and a battered old cooker with a working oven and one plate.

Our little house was quickly beginning to look like a home.

The floors of the house had been in the most terrible condition with nails sticking out of the floorboards and splintered wood. David and I had finally given up hope of doing these repairs and the '*jobs worth*'s at the council said it was my problem, not theirs, they had done all they were *obliged* to do. So I spent the last £200 of my grant having the whole house carpeted. For £200 you can imagine the quality but carpet is carpet and the kindly man who had turned up from the suppliers, with hopes of making thousands of pounds from me, quickly sussed our situation and threw in some underlay and fancy door treads. I am constantly amazed at the kindness people show complete strangers and this man took his place on my own private roll of honour when he had fitted a slightly better quality carpet onto the lounge floor, not to my taste and it clashed most dreadfully with the suite and luxury curtains but did I care? I most certainly did not!

This was just one of so many acts of kindness shown to me over the next few years of my life, kindnesses which would touch my heart and humble me.

During moments of dark despair, I would read a beautiful poem Kate had found and lovingly copied and placed in a frame. One of the few things I miraculously still had. It read:

Footprints

One night I dreamed a dream. I was walking along the beach with my Lord. Across the dark sky flashed scenes from my life. For each scene, I noticed two sets of footprints in the sand, one belonging to me and one to my Lord.

When the last scene of my life flashed before me, I looked back at the footprints in the sand. I noticed that many times along the path of my life there was only one set of footprints. I also noticed that it happened at the very lowest and saddest times of my life.

This really bothered me and I questioned the LORD about it. LORD you said that once I decided to follow you, you'd walk with me all the way. But I have noticed that during the most troublesome times in my life there is only one set of footprints. I don't understand why when I needed you most you would leave me.

The LORD replied, my precious, precious child, I Love you and I would never leave you! During your times of trial and suffering when you see only one set of footprints, it was then that I carried you.

143

Spending the last of my grant on carpets meant all we had to live on from June until October was the family allowance, just £26 a week. I had a card machine fitted for the electricity and put in £5 a week. Fortunately we didn't need coal. I caught the bus to work and we ate Soya mince – so much of it the smell now turns my stomach. I would soak it in herbs overnight and made Soya everything. I could write a book on *100 ways of cooking Soya*. The children often ate at friends' houses and there were one or two free meals at work if I waited tables all day. When visitors came they would always bring food with them, rather than eat anything I might put in front of them, so the summers weren't too bad.

The winters were really hard, but with my grant and student loan we had plenty of food, and I once found the children standing hand in hand in front of the open fridge-freezer – another gift from a friend – staring at the provisions inside in wonder.

Coping with the cold was a real problem. The coal fire central heating with only four radiators barely took the chill off the house and the bathroom was freezing.

I splashed out on the plastic you could heat seal using a hairdryer and covered all the windows. The plastic would bulge terrifyingly when there was the slightest breeze outside, proving how bad the window frames were. Although it helped quite a bit, we were still cold.

In desperation, I asked for a quote for storage heaters, I only needed five to warm the rooms without radiators.

I laughed at the final figure and apologised for wasting the time of the salesman from the electricity board.

Two days later we found two huge storage heaters complete with bricks outside the backdoor of the house and an old heated towel rail. David read out a note left with them.

Mrs Cunningham, hope these help to hold back the cold, put one at the foot of the stairs and one at the top for best service, I will pop round and wire in the towel rail on Saturday morning, if that is convenient.

The storage heaters are in perfect working order, the owner just found them too ugly and has gone for slim line. She gave permission for you to have them and threw in the towel rail.

Ed

"How do you do it mum?" David asked grinning.

"I have no idea," I replied. "But I think it's less of what I do and more about how kind and thoughtful others are."

On this occasion I may have been wrong.

True to his word, Ed arrived early on the Saturday morning and wired in the towel rail.

He didn't get the date with me he asked for – remembering my celibacy oath I wasn't even tempted by a Chinese meal with wine – instead I claimed to be far too busy with work and uni but he did get a sandwich and a cup of tea.

For the first time we were really warm, the heat from the storage heater on the landing warmed my bedroom too and for the first time I could escape there for solitude and the chance to read my ever increasing pile of academic books.

My days as a student were drawing to a close. I'll admit I had found studying very hard and although I sailed through essays – once I had learned to write academically instead of following the rules of journalism – I still found exams a real problem and every year I had re-sits.

With the support of tutors and fellow students I managed to pass each one of these and had my fingers crossed for at least a third because a pass would not give me the honours I had worked so hard for.

On results day I caught the bus to Keele – even if I didn't have a lot to celebrate I was damn sure I was going to celebrate my friends' results, some of whom were almost certainly going to get a first.

I took my time walking to the Chancellor's Building where my friends and I had agreed to meet and check our results. I was so nervous. It had been three long years and a lot of sacrifice and trauma. More than anybody, more than myself, I didn't want to let down David and Louise who had been forced to make this journey with me.

YOU DON'T KNOW WHAT IT'S LIKE

I stood at the top of the steps looking down at the mad, excited throng packed around the notice board.
Right at the front were two of my best friends, Sally and Sylv. Sally spotted me and shouted,
"Babs what did you get?"
"I don't know yet," I laughed "But I bet you know!"
Many other familiar faces were now turned to mine and crossed fingers were held in the air, then …

"A 2:2! You got a 2:2!" shouted Sally with a wide grin on her face. There was a huge roar of applause and I was grabbed and cuddled and hugged and kissed. Sally and Sylvia fought their way to me and the three of us, each with 2:2's, held onto each other and jumped around like children.
"God you are so popular," said Sylvia, everyone including librarians and tutors have been stopping us and asking how you have done.
I was dumb struck! I just couldn't believe it – I had a 2nd class dual honours degree in Criminology and Psychology!
"You are going to have a drink with us aren't you Babs?" shouted Beverly from the middle of the crowd.
"Have a drink with you?" I shouted back. "You'll have to break my fingers to get the bottle away," I laughed.
The rest of the day was a blur of parties and music and celebrations. We sat on the bank in the beautiful gardens of Keele Hall drinking wine straight from the bottle and watching students try

to race across the lake before their home made boats sunk.

I rushed home to change, only having time to cuddle David and Louise and tell them the good news and to phone Kate who nearly exploded down the phone in excitement.

Then back to Keele to enjoy the fun of a fair, hastily erected on the student union car park and to go to endless department discos and cocktail parties.

We partied the night away and I finally fell into bed, a little worse for ware, at about 4 in the morning. At 4.05 the children jumped into bed with me and we sang,

"Mummy got a 2:2, mummy got a 2:2" at the top of our voices until one by one our voices trailed away and we slept.

Job done!!

GRADUATION AND DISAPPOINTMENT

Graduation day dawned and the house was a hive of excitement. The three people I loved most in the world were going to be with me, Kate having arrived the night before.   David and Louise suddenly looking so grown up, David now 16, so handsome in a smart green sports jacket, white shirt, red, green and gold striped tie, beige trousers and brown leather shoes and Louise, 13, looked so pretty in a pale blue dress, blue suede shoes and a cream suede designer jacket sent to her from Germany by my sister Lesley.

I had dug out my 'all occasions' black skirt but had scraped enough money together to buy a new white blouse and black suede shoes and there had been just enough for a pair of black trousers and three-quarter length black velvet jacket for the Graduation Ball in the evening.

Kate looked fabulous in a cream pin striped trouser suit and chocolate brown shirt and planned to wear a cream sparkly top with the trousers in the evening.

Graduation ceremonies had been going on all day, BA's in the morning and my ceremony for BSc's in the afternoon. I stood in front of the mirror, in the packed gymnasium, frowning at the black mortarboard pinned to my thick blonde hair that appeared to be fighting for its freedom, long black gown and gold cape trimmed in red, which refused to stay straight on my inadequate shoulders. What *did* I look like? Then I grinned back at my reflection ... I looked like a Keele University

Graduate, that's what I looked like … and walked happily out into the hot sunshine with my friends to the university chapel where our ceremony was to be held.

I entered the chapel as plain Barbara Cunningham and exited as *Barbara Cunningham BSc!!!*

I began to despair when, in the next few weeks, I had applied for at least 20 jobs and not received a single reply. I was nearly 50 and became convinced my age was going against me as all my younger friends had found jobs, although some were going on to study for Masters and PhD's. The plan had been to return to Essex when I graduated, but David and Louise were settled in good schools and doing so well, I felt moving them again would be unfair, so I was forced to look for work in Staffordshire alone.

In the end I turned to Keele Careers Advice for help. They suggested I attach a photograph to any further applications.

"They need to see how attractive you are and how young you look," I was told.

So I had to 'look young and attractive,' I thought sadly as I walked back to my car.

"For a 2:2 graduate you look depressed," said a cheerful voice. "We checked you out on results day," laughed Mary from Human Resources. "Well done I bet you are thrilled."

I had got to know Mary and her colleagues when I was looking for work whilst studying and they had found me the job in the Hawthorns Restaurant on campus.

"I would be if I could get a job," I told her despondently.

Mary told me there was a vacancy in Keele Library.

"It's semesters only, paid over 12 months but could keep you going until something better comes up," she said.

"Anything," I said, throwing my arms around her and planting a big kiss on her rosy cheek.

We walked arm in arm back to her department in Keele Hall to complete an application form and within three weeks I started work in the Nuffield Library where I had spent so many hours studying and vowed, when I graduated, I wouldn't step foot in again.

Many books in heavy demand, mainly course work, are kept in the Nuffield Library. The majority of these books are on short loan and incur heavy fines when returned late.

This was the busiest part of the library, the part where tears were shed and tempers lost when students came back, over and over again, only to find some rich, thoughtless student was hanging on to the copy they had reserved.

Although not the job of my dreams it was actually very convenient. I was home for the school holidays and could find other work to make a little more money during vacations.

Most of all I enjoyed the work. It was hard and tiring, occasionally boring, but I enjoyed the interaction with the students and academics from all over the world and I was still enjoying a love affair with Keele and its beautiful surroundings and I had not yet tired of Staffordshire.

In some ways, I was the 'librarian from hell' often being told good-naturedly by the students to 'shush' but I was good at my job and popular with the students, often lending them my own books, or if they were studying my subjects, recommending readings and texts.

On the whole I got on with other members of staff calling them 'The Ladies of the Library' but it was here, however, that I had my first experience of being bullied and what a shock to my system that was.

Her name was Sadie, 'Shady Sadie' I liked to call her behind her back. She was a thin, blonde 24 year old, quite pretty, intelligent, hard working and a Keele English graduate but she was also spoiled, spiteful and suffering from a serious case of 'Babs Envy.'

Things were really OK between us to begin with. She was a grade above me and therefore worked all year round. She had a great sense of humour and was capable of making me giggle helplessly with her quick wit and gift of telling a tale about some experience or the other.

However, her life had been very sheltered. She had lived at home with her parents whilst a student at Keele and, unlike most young students, had missed the fun of living in halls. Even now she was driven to work by her father, picked up at lunchtime, fed and returned and picked up again in the evening. She didn't have a social life and everything she did was with her mother and father, occasionally visiting her sister who was married to an airman and living in the south somewhere.

The problems started when she announced she was leaving. She was moving with her parents to be nearer her sister who had three children and 'needed support' when her husband was away.

I applied successfully for her job and on my first day in that position she announced that their house sale had fallen through and that she was staying at Keele. To her utter humiliation, she was told the only vacancy available was my old job, making me now senior to her.

From that point on things became very, very different.

Why did I let it happen? You may well ask and I am not sure I can come up with an answer. I can only speculate that, as I had never been bullied before, I simply didn't recognise it for what it was.

Sadie was unrelenting. It would start first thing in the morning. It was our job to open the Nuffield at the start of the day. This was done in absolute silence, apart from her sighing and tutting, often doing my job and not hers, and she would arrive earlier and earlier in order for that to happen.

She often had lengthy whispered conversations on the phone with her mother, whom she had only left a few minutes ago, with SHE being the only audible word as she threw a scathing look in my direction.

She would comment in front of others on the speed I worked, the way I worked, my relationship with the students and staff. She would notice every tiny error I made and report it and if I dared bite back, she would run from the library in floods of tears seeking solace on the shoulder of anyone who could be bothered to give her airtime. For Sadie was not popular and the Ladies of the Library, indeed the men too, were very well aware of whom the troublemaker was.

I turned to my managers for support and when that failed I went to Michael, the Head Librarian.

He called us both in for a 'little' chat and then told us to try and work together, suggesting we shook hands. With heavy heart, but willing to give it a try, I held my hand out to Sadie, wanting all the problems to end. She ignored it and simply said to Michael,

"I'm not shaking hands with her," and stomped out of his office.

"Try to work with her Babs," Michael pleaded, "Or just ignore her."

Anyone who has been in that position knows how difficult it is to ignore someone who is making your life a misery.

My Achilles heel was finally breached one morning when only she and I were in the Nuffield. Sadie came in with a huge spider in a jar and now smiling for once she shoved it under my nose and asked me what type of spider I though it was.

YOU DON'T KNOW WHAT IT'S LIKE

I have always suffered from arachnophobia and any size spider can make me feel physically sick and leave me whimpering in uncontrolled fear. We had had several spiders in the Nuffield and my fear had always been taken seriously and with some sympathy, when others told of their own phobias.

I fled from the Nuffield in total panic and was found sometime later, cowering in the ladies loo, by Rose, one of my managers.

"We knew you were here," she said putting her arm around me, "What on earth is the matter?"

Still shaking and tearful I told her about the spider.

"The bitch," said Rose. "I'll deal with this. You go home and don't come back until tomorrow."

'Tomorrow' took three months as my body gave way to what I realised much later was a deep and dark depression – everything, all the past sadness and trauma seemed to implode on me.

I found it hard to get out of bed in the morning and struggled to get off the sofa and away from the television during the day.

As usual, I gave pretence of normality when the children were around, but behind their backs I slept and was forced to dash around tidying and cleaning in a panic, half an hour before they came home from school.

I went to the Doctors complaining of various maladies – bad back, painful knees and foot, which were true … ish! Mysterious headaches and stomach-aches – if it existed, I had it in those three months.

One day, sitting in the doctor's surgery yet again, a light suddenly came on in my head.

Depression! I nearly leapt to my feet for I had suddenly worked out what was wrong with me – I was suffering from depression. So much for the doctors who had sent me for blood tests and urine tests and every test under the sun, but so much for me too – as a psychology graduate it should have come to me sooner.

I almost skipped into the doctor's office …

"I've diagnosed myself," I grinned. "Don't need you anymore. I'm suffering from depression."

I started back at work the following Monday. I noticed with satisfaction the dismay on Sadie's face, when the afternoon break included chocolate and fruit cake and a large bottle of wine – my colleagues had been busy cooking in preparation of celebrating my return.

I felt so good, so happy to be back to my old self. Just one little job left to do.

At the end of the late night Sadie and I worked together, in silence as usual, but it didn't bother me as I had the company of the students and other staff to enjoy. I waited for her at the bottom of the steps to the library. Taking her by surprise, I grabbed hold of her and pinned her skinny little body to the wall, my arm under her chin.

"Don't you ever think of even trying to bully me again you little shit," I hissed into her shocked face.

"You do and I will sue the arse off you, your mother, your poor old taxi driver and every bloody spider in your house!!"

I let go of her but as I turned to walk away, brushing my hands together in an exaggerated theatrical style, I shouted back at her,

"And don't bother reporting this, after all, who would *ever* believe you." As I threw her an angelic smile I heard shouts from one of the many library windows ...

"Way to go Babs!"

"You sure showed her Babs!"

"Blimey duck, yer little but tough!" – followed by a round of applause, laughter and whistling.

I felt a little ashamed of my behaviour as I climbed into my battered old car, after all violence, I knew to my cost, solves nothing. 'Oh well,' I thought, 'I'll just have to learn to live with it' ... and chuckled.

THE INTERNET WORLD
Grapevine 50's

I had no further problems with Shady Sadie and the years rolled by, uneventful years. I was aware that most of the library staff had been there all their working lives, in fact I found the thought quite frightening that I might stay there, for the rest of my working life, stamping books and shelving them.

I became restless, constantly asking for more interesting work but as nobody left there was little or no chance of promotion.

Recognising my frustration and wasted abilities, the library Director, Richard, seconded me to the Admissions Department for the summer vacation.

I was thrilled to bits, the work was varied and interesting, I dealt mainly with foreign student applications but was also involved with open days and showing hopeful students and their families around the university and of course the mania of 'clearing.'

Clearing is the rush for remaining places by prospective students who had failed to be accepted by the universities of their first choice. It was an emotional and difficult time for them – and for us, it meant thinking on our feet, making snap decisions based on telephone interviews with pleading hopefuls not at their best due to their desperation.

I loved it and I worked hard, hoping that I might be able to remain part of this department at the end of my secondment.

YOU DON'T KNOW WHAT IT'S LIKE

As usual, fate stepped in and changed the course of my life.

One lunchtime, as I was walking across the field to the university store, a football came bouncing toward me.

"Over here, Babs," shouted a fresh-faced PhD student I recognised from the chemistry department. He and several other students were having a celebratory game of football having just handed in their theses.

Not respecting my age – I was now 52 – and arthritic body – a throwback to too many years of playing netball – I joined in the game with gusto and I wasn't bad (I still tell the tale of the goal I scored from 25 yards outside the area.) I wasn't bad, that is, until my foot went down a hole and I fell, cracking the already crumbling cartilage in my kneecap.

X-rays showed I needed an operation and I was put on the waiting list. I was told I would be waiting for at least 9 months.

I thought I would go out of my mind. I was trapped, I couldn't work, I couldn't drive, I had few friends as most of them had scattered after graduating and I was 200 miles away from my Essex pals. The children, now both in their teens, were hardly at home. I had to find something non-active to do, something to fill the days. Then Louise came up with an idea she thought would be amusing ... she put me in an internet chat room for people in their 50's. Suddenly I had all the company I needed to fill my days and, at times, my sleepless nights and the nickname Lou gave me was the name she'd given me as a child … BIONICBABS.

I sat mesmerized staring at the screen, I was in a 'room' called *Grapevine 50's* and there were over 60 people all typing at the same time and yet knowing what conversation they were part of or which individual they were chatting to.
As the screen scrolled at a terrifying pace I noticed a few had greeted my arrival, there was a mixture of …
"Hi Babs."
"Hi BB."
"Hello bionic."
"BionicBabs, welcome xx."
"BionicBabs … you new?"
But by the time I had raised my hands to type a reply, the screen had scrolled on and their nicknames were lost in the ether.
I decided to sit and watch this fascinating new world go by, unable as yet to keep up.
Even here there appeared to be protocols: you greeted people as they *entered* and they said 'hi' in return and you bade them 'farewell' when they were leaving, you didn't *'whisper'* without first asking for permission from the member you wanted to have a private conversation with, although I soon learned this was not strictly adhered to.

The room was controlled by *Bots*, robotic thingies – sorry to those techies reading this – and *Hosts*, real ladies, drinking coffee. They monitored the room and kicked out people using abusive language but seemed to miss those just being abusive! It didn't make much difference, these odd balls tended just to change their nicknames and re-enter to carry on with the abuse.

There were also short forms to learn, for example …

Wb, *welcome back,*

lol, *laughs out loud,*

rofl, *rolls on floor laughing,*

pmsl, meant – oh very nice – *piss myself laughing,*

lmfao, *laugh my fat arse off,* I didn't use that one – would never admit to that part of my anatomy being anything other than pert.

There was wit and humour used in 'chat', and incredible sadness disclosed. People were angry, lonely, sad, depressed and bitter. It was a little world some took far too seriously and to some it was their *only* world, a world where they could pretend to be anything and everything they had ever dreamed of being.

There were 'room bullies' who used large, brash coloured fonts. They would totally dominate conversations, demand attention and insult anyone who disagreed or challenged them. These few would often enter 'mob handed' having phoned their friends first and timed their entrance. I had visions of children being rushed to school, hastily taken coffee breaks, shopping put off until later and washing lying wet in laundry baskets whilst outside the sun shone brightly. These few could empty the chat room in 10 minutes, with only their loyal supporters remaining and those wanting to become part of the 'gang' for safety sake, and me, wondering how the hell they got away with it and had been for years, for they often said,

'I have been coming in here for four years, since this room opened.' What pleasure did it give them and when would my day come to take them on?

I was a quick learner and soon became accepted as a regular *chatter* in the room. It was a great medium for me and brought back to life the writing skills that had lain dormant for so long, and this was such fun. I found I loved writing with humour and there were few, if any, who could take me on in a written battle. I earned a reputation as a fighter, taking up the gauntlet for those less capable of defending themselves and in turn was often picked on by the room bullies but hey, I wasn't going to be bullied again in the real world let alone in a chat room!

It wasn't long before I realised chatters had published profiles and photographs, you simply had to 'click' on their nicknames and there it was, a nice big photograph. What a shock that was! I couldn't quite get my head around *cutelittlebunnyrabbit* being an 18 stone woman with thick horn rimmed glasses and a blue rinse in her tightly permed hair or *melgibson05* being of equal size but with no hair. Many of the women had pretty suggestive names like *peekaboobra* and *prettylacestockingtops6*, there were several *gorgeousblonde's* and *bustybabe's*. The chat room was full of *angels* and *fairies* and they were in competition with *teacher*, *nursey*, *sexymum* and a sprinkling of *sexygrans*.

The men selected far more macho nicknames – there were quite a few cars – *mercman*, *66BMW66*, *breadrollsroyce*, a selection of *motorbikes*, then there were *boxers*, *wrestlers* and *fighters* and to my great joy, having always had a weakness for men in uniform, *soldiers* and *airmen*, *pilots* and *police*. Sadly, *Berttheretiredplumber* was nearer the truth, for when I stole a peek at their photographs, many of the men in the 50's chat room looked more like my dad!

It was the first time since my school days that I found myself interacting with my own peer group in any great numbers. My life thus far had been filled with younger friends, at netball, at college, even at university – all my friends were at the very least 8 years younger than I was. My self-imposed celibacy now meant I was trapped in a time warp. It had been 10 years since I had last done any meaningful flirting and sadly I seemed to still be attracted to men 10 years younger than I was, if not more. But then, I wasn't in chat to meet men, I was in chat-to-chat.

"Why no pic Babs?" I was often asked.
"Cos I'm dead ugly," was my usual reply.
The truth was I had lost a lot of confidence in my appearance. If I was shocked at the pictures of

others I chatted to, why wouldn't they be shocked when they saw a picture of me?

In the end I bit the bullet and published a photograph taken on my cheap cam. It was a little fuzzy but it was definitely me, grinning out from under a mass of long dark hair.

The reaction was astonishing, adoration and praise and proposals of marriage from some men, mixed with snide, ugly and abusive comments from others. There was hatred, bitterness and spite from many of the women, some claimed the picture was not of me, it was taken 20 years ago, women of my age shouldn't have long hair and what the hell was a woman like me doing in a chat room?

The picture stayed, it gave me plenty of new material, new battles to be won in *grapevine 50's* and I made many friends, some who became friends in the real world, who didn't give a stuff what I looked like. They liked me and that was all that mattered.

REDREDWINE

It was the early hours of the morning. My knee was agony so I hobbled down stairs and turned on the pc. I clicked onto *Grapevine 50's* to see if there was anyone still awake to play with and as my old computer groaned and hummed into life I limped into the kitchen to pour myself a fair sized brandy – purely for medicinal purposes you understand.

Back at the pc I was surprised to see the chat room still buzzing. There were about 30 people in chatting and I had missed quite a few 'hi Babs.'

They seemed to recognise each other although many of the nicknames were new to me. I assumed these were people who worked late and this was their early evening. There appeared to be some sort of argument going on with others taking sides. 'Great,' I thought, settling back, my brandy cuddled to my chest, 'Maybe I can join in once I know what's going on.'

It wasn't a fight, it was a man nicknamed *Redredwine* begging *silverhairedlady* for forgiveness. 'Wow what's he done?' I wondered. 'A two timing rat? An affair? He stood her up? Must be something really, really bad.'

I thought it was hilarious when I discovered he had fallen asleep at his pc whilst chatting to her in whisper the night before.

Most were on his side so I decided to go into bat for the lady.

Redredwine: *I'm so sorry lady please forgive me*

Silverhairedlady   *someone tell him he's blocked*
BionicBabs: *Red you're blocked*
Ktypmsl: *awww go on lady he's so sorry*
Purdy: *Go on lady, red's such a nice fella*
BionicBabs: *Don't you lady, make him suffer lol*
Ktypmsl: *Babs!!!* (I loved *kty* she was the sweetest lady in chat)
Wilma: *what're you lot doin up* (Wilma, another daytime friend of mine who became a friend in the real world)
BionicBabs: *Hi Wilms, we're making Red sweat!!*
Wilms: *Trust you Babs it's that knee of yours makin you feisty*
BionicBabs: *I think his knees should hurt, he should be down on them!!*

A little orange light started to flash at the bottom of my screen. Oh dear, here we go, it was *Redredwine* wanting to whisper.
"Hello my name is Tony."
"Hi Tone," I replied dubiously.
"You're a good looking woman Babs," he wrote to my surprise.
"Naah just clever wiv me makeup," I replied.
As the room scrolled by we chatted on. I took a quick look at his picture and was pleasantly surprised to find he had hair and a waist.
Silverhairedlady: (proving she hadn't blocked *Redredwine* because she'd noticed his absence from the room conversation), *where's the rat gone now, I bet he's asleep again*

"Your girlfriend is looking for you," I pointed out to Tony.

"Much rather chat to you," he wrote.

"She's gorgeous … I took a quick look at her pic."

She was indeed a stunning looking woman, the same age as myself, not a wrinkle or puffy bit in sight.

"Air brushed," wrote Tony.

"I beg your pardon?"

"Her pics. She paid over £100 for them, they've been airbrushed, she doesn't look anything like that in real life. Fancy a coffee sometime? I'm close by, in Wales, but I work in Cheshire."

Whoops, with that I switched off the pc, didn't even bother to shut down correctly and limped back to bed taking my half drunk glass of brandy with me.

It was about time I sat down and had a talk with myself. I was alone again for the weekend. David and Louise often spent the weekends with friends in town, living in a village with a limited bus service was simply not convenient when everything was 'happening' half an hour away.

I didn't mind I was pleased they had friends and a social life and both of them were continually on the phone, checking up on their mum. As if I ever got up to anything!

I had to admit I was feeling very lonely. Friends had always surrounded me but now I occasionally had visits from colleagues and then they had husbands and children in tow and of course Kate

167

came up as often as she could but that was really only three or four times a year. I missed her dreadfully and my knee stopped me driving to Essex. I had to do something, I needed a social life!

I was still having fun in '50s' and was learning to flirt again – in fact it had come back to me quite easily really!

Redredwine: *Did you crash last night Babs*
BionicBabs: *errrr no, I mean yes, no I mean no*
Ace: *did she do a runner Red, you must have asked her out*
RichMe: *did a runner when I asked her out*
Waveydavey: I *never asked her out, heard she did a runner lol*
BionicBabs: *Oiiiiiii you guys I am here ya know*
Redredwine: *How about that coffee Babs*
BionicBabs: *what coffee?*
Redredwine: *last night, I mentioned meeting for coffee*
BionicBabs: *don't remember I was doin a runner lol*

Tony took our conversation into whisper.
"Hey Babs, it's just coffee or a drink in a pub of your choice, nothing more, just two chat room friends meeting up."
"OK Tone," good grief what had I just typed, too late I had pressed *enter.*
"WOW great, Thursday any good, I have Thursday evening off?"

YOU DON'T KNOW WHAT IT'S LIKE

With my heart in my mouth I agreed to Thursday evening. I even agreed to him picking me up from home.

"I won't invite you in Tone, just sound your horn and I'll hobble out, I don't have a stick so you will have to offer me your arm to lean on haha."

"If you look anything like your pic I will be proud to have you on my arm," wrote Tony.

I shut down the computer before I got myself into any more grief, it was only Sunday night and I was already in a panic.

"I don't want to go," I wailed, "I'm too old for this dating stuff."

"Oh shush mum," said Lou, "You're on your own too much, you're getting boring," she laughed.

Lou was sitting on my bed whilst David leant against my bedroom door looking concerned.

"You do intend introducing this man to me don't you?" he asked sombrely.

I laughed.

"You sound like my dad. No I'm not bringing him in, we're just going for a drink and then I'm coming straight home, that's it."

"But what do you know about this man?" David asked, obviously quite concerned about my impending tryst, "I mean, a *chat room* mum, after everything you have read in the papers about chat rooms."

I turned to look at my son's sweet worried face. Lou stood up and put her arms around his neck.

"Aww he's being the daddy again," she teased. But I knew she was trying to pacify the brother she adored.

"I'll NEVER be like him," David said truculently.

"Look David, it's not perfect, I'll grant you that," I said. "But I don't have the option of meeting someone in a pub or club or at work or even in ASDA and a 50's chat room is not quite like rooms children go in to. If I can't take care of myself, after all these years and everything I have been through, well I may as well lie down and die." I limped over to my two wonderful children and we had a group hug and I felt so very small, they were now both taller than me … how time flies.

"Well don't be late back," David said, smiling down at me, "Or I won't trust you out on your own again."

I understood perfectly how strange this must be to David and Lou, there had only ever been their father and Jim in my life and Lou had been too young to even recall her father being around. Oh, I'd been out alright and had some really wild times but in groups, never, in 10 years, on my own with a man.

"Right, how do I look?" I asked, attempting a twirl, showing off the cream, pinstriped trouser suit I had inherited from Kate.

"Stunning mum," said David.

"Very bionic," said Lou with a knowing grin.

"Well as long as I look like my pic I won't fall over," I laughed – then waved my hand to dismiss the statement when I noticed their puzzled frowns …

"I'll explain later."

With that they both carefully helped me down the stairs and a very stubborn David helped me down the path to Tony's waiting, spotlessly clean, bright red Rover.

They shook hands and I laughed when David said, "Look after her," and Tony, the image of his photograph, promised he would. He climbed into the driver's seat next to me and just before pulling away he leaned across and gave me a peck on the cheek and said,

"You're one good looking woman, Babs, I'm going to be so proud to have you on my arm."

I breathed a sigh of relief. 'A good looking woman' he had said. Maybe I can still cut it in the real world. So far so good!

I couldn't have wished for a better first date. Tony was such a nice man. I didn't get flowers or chocolates, I got a rather attractive hospital walking stick he had dug out having abandoned it many years before when he no longer needed it.

He was polite, caring and attentive. He was also a graduate from Keele so we instantly had something in common. Although he had been there many years before me not much had changed.

One of the things I liked most about him was that his caring highlighted when I had a *power surge*. OK, OK, a hot flush – the menopause rolled on! He went outside with me, put plastic down on a bench and sat with me in the pouring rain holding a large golf umbrella over my head until the sweats disappeared and my colour returned to normal. Of course I was then chilled and shivered. He then removed his jacket, wrapped it around my shoulders until the next power surge gripped my totally exhausted body.

There was no chemistry on my part, although Tony made it quite clear there was on his. This didn't bother me at all. I was out, I was on a date and I was going to take little tiny steps in my brave new world.

We talked endlessly about the chat room. I was fascinated. Tony had been using it for four years. He was a self-employed taxi driver and used it when he got home late at night to help him wind down.

He had met several people at *meets* – social occasions when everyone got together – and he had also dated several women from *50's* and indeed from *40's* where he was also a member.

"Few look anything like their pictures," he told me, "In fact the majority don't and their profiles are pure fantasy."

"A woman I met from the *40's* must have been in her 60's and admitted using a photograph of her daughter."

I was quite shocked and a little disappointed but he boldly told me I was rather naïve.

"Many people in chat lack self esteem, are shy or damaged in some way. They use chat rooms because they can be anything they want to be – well they could years ago when you couldn't download an image."

"They came unstuck with the publishing of photographs," he continued. "Having described themselves for years as slim blonde and beautiful they were suddenly forced to find photographs that portrayed them in that way."

"But why do they meet people when they know they look nothing like their pictures?" I asked, hoping this wise man had the answer.

"For some it's their whole world, they have no other life," he replied. "They get swept up in the lie and actually believe it. I did actually tell one woman that her photograph was very flattering – of course I was being sarcastic – but she thanked me," he laughed.

"I'm so glad you look like your pics," he grinned.

"And I you," I said frowning, wondering what the hell I would have done if a hobbit had climbed out of the bright red Rover.

I was home by 11.15, much to the relief of 'the daddy' and his sister who were standing by the window as we drew up but scattered immediately and were calmly sitting watching the television when I entered the lounge. They were full of questions and disappointed when I told them we had sat in the rain talking about Keele and chat rooms.

I knew they were happy when I told them I was going to see Tony again and even happier, I do believe, when I told them there was no chemistry and he wouldn't be moving in anytime soon, we were just friends.

My dating Tony awakened my children's curiosity about their father. Since we had been in the

Midlands they hadn't heard from him, not a card or a phone call, although he knew our address and telephone numbers at all times. I had heard that he had consulted a solicitor in an attempt to stop me going to university but was told that he had no chance of succeeding as I was trying to improve the children's and my situation and he gave me no money toward their upbringing. It had shown, yet again, that this was more about Bob's desire to control me rather than stay close to his children.

As I sat at my dressing table, removing the makeup from my face, David and Lou came in and sprawled across my bed, as they so often did when a little bit stressed.

"Was he always bad?" Lou asked, never one to pull her punches. I knew she was talking about Bob.

"He was a boozer wasn't he mum?" said David who, after so many years, still missed having his father in his life.

"Yes he was," I replied, fighting to remain honest on this sensitive subject, "But he really did try to stop and he did succeed for a while."

BOB: A REASON NOT AN EXCUSE

Bob had been a drinker for many years, like his father before him who had died an alcoholic. He had tried really hard to stop when we met and had succeeded for a number of years but he had gradually returned to it when our first baby was stillborn and he had to watch me give birth, at full term, to our lifeless little girl.

I had been worried all through this first pregnancy. I looked and felt ill and at nearly nine months, I started to be violently sick every time I moved. At the anti-natal clinic I would watch other mother's wombs move as their unborn babies kicked and turned but I would only feel slight flutters first thing in the morning and then, with time, nothing. On a scheduled visit to my Doctor I told him of my concerns, but he had simply told me I was a 'worrying mother' and that he had heard the baby's heart beating. He did say, however, that he was worried about my blood pressure and that I had sugar in my urine sample. This, he explained, showed early signs of toxaemia, blood poisoning in pregnancy and he had sent me home to rest for a week.

The nightmare began on my next visit when he failed to find a foetal heartbeat and told me he thought the baby had probably died. I had to drive home, on my own. I had to phone Bob who worked in London and wait two hours for him to get home. Both of us then drove in torment to the local maternity hospital in Braintree where my womb was scanned for signs of life ... again, nothing. From there we were sent to St John's Hospital in Chelmsford, both of us weeping on that terrible journey. I was scanned again and this time we were told that there was no doubt. Our baby was dead.

The horror continued when I was told it was better for me if I gave birth naturally and they also wanted me to hold my child. I was horrified, screamed *I couldn't do that* but they simply promised me I would feel no pain. Because the baby was dead they could pump me full of drugs – drugs that would have cost a fortune on the black market.

Bob stayed by my side throughout and when she was born I begged to hold her and we broke our hearts over the body of our tiny child who weighed less than 2 lbs.

One nurse had stayed with me throughout, calmly and quietly performing her duties and long after Bob had gone she stayed with me and held me until finally, exhausted, I fell asleep.

I can't remember much of that dreadful night in hospital, except for waking in a room of my own and hearing the distant screams of the pain of mothers giving birth and the crying of healthy babies, whilst my lifeless child lay in a crib at the foot of my bed. I was too weak to reach out and hold her and in the morning she was gone.

In the weeks that followed, I had put Bob through agony begging him to try to draw the little face I couldn't remember and he tried, although it was breaking his heart, he really tried.

And then I learned that the hospital took photos of stillborn babies, dressed and lying in a crib as if asleep, but more pain was to follow when I was told that the practice was new, so new that it was not carried out when I had had my baby.

At that time I was also told that the government paid for all stillborn babies to be placed in their own little coffins and buried locally on a plot reserved especially for all children who had died. I was advised to contact the Stillbirth Association who would help me find where my child was buried.

This gave me hope for I needed a place to go, somewhere to visit to grieve over my child.

A kindly lady visited me from the Association who told me it would take just two weeks to obtain the information I needed … but life was to deal me yet another mean blow.

She returned within two weeks, pail and sombre faced. She asked if Bob was home and when I said no, she suggested she came back when he was. I couldn't wait and pressed her for any information she had.

"Mrs Cunningham, I have such bad news," she said. "The undertaker responsible for the burial of your baby was, how can I put this, 'fiddling the books'. He claimed money for, as far as we can tell 9 coffins, but instead was placing the babies in the coffins of adults."

She came and sat beside me and took my hands in hers.

"He committed suicide a few weeks ago and burned all his records first. Through a process of elimination, based on time and dates, we were able to locate the burial sites of all but two of the babies. I am so sorry but one of those two was your little girl."

After she was gone I phoned Bob but all he could hear was my hysteria, he couldn't make out my words or understand the problem.

Sick with worry he rushed home to find me totally traumatised, just saying over and over again,

"She's lost, our baby is lost."

He called a doctor who gave me something to make me sleep and then he held me all through the night, comforting me when I cried out in pain.

It wasn't until the following afternoon, that I was able to tell him the horrible news from the Association and then it was my turn to hold him whilst he cried.

It was shortly after that – I later discovered – that Bob started to drink again.

David was born 12 months later on *exactly* the same day and in the same room as our lifeless little baby had been born and although he was perfect, he was 5 weeks early and very tiny. At that time, I was unable to see this incredible coincidence as the hand of God offering me, in a kind, loving way, a 'replacement' for the baby I had lost. David's birthday would always remind me of the loss of my little girl. To me it was a cruel twist of fate.

I was told he needed to go into the Special Care Baby Unit (SCUBU) as he was jaundiced and needed specialist treatment. For the first few days after his birth David's liver did not work as well as it should. There was a build-up of bilirubin in his blood. This caused his skin and the whites of his eyes to turn yellow.

I was informed that, in the human body, new blood is being made all the time and old blood is being destroyed. One of the products of destroyed blood is called bilirubin. Bilirubin normally goes to the liver to be processed and then leaves the body in the faeces. In David's case this was not happening.

The treatment necessary was to place him naked, with a protective mask over his eyes, rather like a meet bag, under a bright light. This, I was told, was called *phototherapy.* The light would break down the bilirubin in his skin and the jaundice would subsequently fade.

David was taken to the nursery in the ward, stripped naked and placed in a crib under lights. It was a frosty November day and as I sat with him I noticed how cold the room was and he seemed to be shivering. I could feel no heat when I placed my hand under these lights and puzzled I went in search of advice from staff in the SCUBU.

"Where is he"? I was asked and when I told them he was in the nursery under the lights all hell broke loose.

"We put them in there to get them out of the way," said an outraged nurse, referring to the lights. "The damn things don't work!!"

David was rushed to the SCUBU, he was now shivering violently.

Sick with worry, I was suddenly aware of the young nurse who had placed him under the lights in the nursery, getting shouted at by a very angry Staff Nurse.

"Didn't you wonder why there were no babies in the nursery?" she was saying. "Not only are the lights faulty but also the heating in there's not working. You could have killed this baby."

Frightened, I looked back at David who had blessedly stopped shivering. The heat in the SCUBU was almost unbearable and at last, although blindfolded, he seemed content and was kicking his tiny yellow legs against the side of the crib.

Bob was horrified when I told him what had happened and shouted in fury and fear at the nurse in charge of the SCUBU.

Later that week, when I returned home, David asleep in my arms, I noticed several empty whiskey bottles on the floor of the lounge. Bob explained that a few of his friends had visited him during the course of the week whilst I was in hospital, bringing with them bottles of whisky to celebrate the birth of his son. I felt reassured when he told me that he had only consumed a couple of glasses.

Nearly three years later Louise was born. Because of the still birth and David's premature arrival, it was decided I should go into hospital early and be induced.

I was determined this birth would go perfectly to order and I would have some control, so as the contractions started I walked around my room singing 'the grand old Duke of York, he had 10,000 men he marched them up to the top of the hill (this was when my pain was at its height) and he marched them down again (relax and breathe).'

A young trainee nurse came into the room and asked if she could feel my tummy.

Happy to oblige I climbed onto my bed and lay back.

"Hmm I can't feel the head," she said frowning. "I'm not very good at this yet I'll get someone to help me."

Within seconds she appeared with a staff Nurse who also failed to feel the head of my baby.

Still unconcerned, I lay back patiently whilst a surgeon poked and prodded my womb.

"It's sideways," he shouted at Staff. "Good God didn't anyone check before she was given the drink?"

"Mrs Cunningham, you can give birth to a baby head first and you can give birth to a baby feet first but you cannot give birth to a baby that is lying sideways and at this stage in your labour it's far too late to try to turn it." With that, I was put on a trolley and rushed to the theatre for an emergency caesarean section.

As the mask was placed over my face, the last thing I heard was Bob shouting angrily in the background. He must have just arrived and been told the bad news.

"You killed the first, you nearly killed the second and now you're trying to fucking kill the third."

Louise was beautiful, a little cold so she was wearing a hat, coat and gloves and lying on her own little electric blanket but she was perfect. One of her arms had been trapped above her head whilst she was in my womb and it wanted to keep springing back there, so a bandage had been wrapped around her tiny torso, pinning the arm to her side.

Bob failed to visit that night and friends later found him lying drunk on the floor of our flat, two empty whiskey bottles beside him.

"That was the beginning of the end really. He didn't try to stop drinking again and spent more and more time away from home." I explained to my children who had listened to the story so quietly, never once interrupting.

"So it was *my* fault," Lou said sadly.

"No, no, no, no," I said worried, climbing onto the bed next to them and pulling both of them close to me.

"*He* was to blame and only he. *His* way of dealing with a problem was to look for the answer at the bottom of a bottle without giving a thought for me and, sadly, without giving a thought for either of you."

"There's plenty of help out there for people with drink problems, as I told him so many, many times, and he always promised he would get help. At the end of the day he *chose* to carry on the way he was and well, you know how it ended."

"He lost something precious because he didn't stop drinking, he lost watching you two wonderful young people grow and evolve to who you are today. I love you both so much and wherever you are you will always have me and you will always have each other."

They kissed me and went off to their bedrooms. I knew they were both sad and that nothing I could ever say or do would completely take away that pain, a pain I would share with them for the rest of my life.

COLIN

Tony and I met on many occasions after that first date. We even met another person, *wildjinny*, from the chat room and the three of us, with our combined knowledge, took part and won a couple of local pub quizzes.
I still wasn't keen on meeting men from the chat room – too many spiteful people used it, thriving on rumour and gossip, and I liked to use it merely for fun. So I decided to look elsewhere on the Internet and joined a couple of dating sites.

These sites are a minefield, not for the faint hearted or vulnerable. There are so many *people* – yes, not only *men* – who use them, ever watchful and ready to exploit the naïve, lonely and innocent.
However, there is no excuse for plain stupidity and it makes my blood boil when a single mother posts photographs of herself and all her children! She need only add 'Paedophiles Apply Here.' Or there are the sadly newly widowed with photographs of themselves posing in their beautifully furnished homes or standing by expensive cars and then they admit they are lonely with no friends or family. I mean dohhhhh, guess who's going to be in touch with you, Mr or Miss 'I can help you invest your money!!'

I joined two sites and published honest photographs and profiles.
My profile read:

YOU DON'T KNOW WHAT IT'S LIKE

BIONICBABS

HEADLINE

Will settle for nothing less than a man who can take my breath away!!

PROFILE

Bit of a renegade 54 year old still wear Doc Martens.
I am 'The Librarian From Hell'!!
I do love my job but it can be stressful, so have my pipe, slippers and a nice cuppa' ready for me when I return home from work (joking about the slippers).
I enjoy sport, although I have to be bribed with a trip to Oxfam and a promise of being able to buy anything I like, if the choice of the day is snooker (yawn).
I enjoy most music, can be seen 'shaking my ass' to rock or equally, lying in a darkened room with my bra over my eyes, listening to Vivaldi.
I love to dance and sing, I used to be a singer with a big band, so I don't sound too bad in the bath!
I am a bubbly extrovert, can hold my own in most debates, as long as I have the comfort of a thesaurus in my bag and have noted all the exits.
OK I'm in my 50's but I find that number represents less of who I am and more about what I have to offer in life experience, knowledge and

diversity (if you believe that you're my kind of man)!!

BionicBabs perfect partner

I would love to meet a man who wants to live his life not mine.
A man who doesn't want to change me, who is warm and sincere and doesn't mistake sarcasm for humour, I want him to know when I'm being sarcastic!!
Someone fit, active and still working, I'm not into couch potatoes.
A man who likes to shop… because I hate it.
A man whose eyes don't glaze over when I rant about what a rotten day I've had but would spare me the details of his rotten day.
Someone who would travel when retired and not feel restricted by bricks and mortar.
A man with his own friends and interests.
Someone I feel comfortable with socially and content with privately.
All the above can be overlooked if you are a wiz in the kitchen and a .... oops what did I nearly say!! (giggle)

Before I knew where I was I had received hundreds of emails from both sites and decided I needed a filtering system. My plan had been to answer every email I received, if people took the time to write to me I could at least find the time to reply to them. This soon changed when I found men could say what they liked on these sites. Foul language, suggestive and down right filthy mail was not checked or monitored by site administrators.

Some I replied to – if I could be bothered to think of an appropriately sarcastic reply, for example:

Mail received from:
ivorhardon:
Hi Babs, mst admit just wanked over your photographs, ure ded sexy, plz add me to MSN xxx

Reply:
BionicBabs:
Sorry, I don't add wankers!

Mail received from:
Sexcsquaddie:
Just used your pictures to masturbate, hope you don't mind

Reply:
BionicBabs:
If ya hands are that rough, knock yaself out

Mail received from:
ToyBoy10:
Hey Babs wanna watch me cum on cam?

Reply:
BionicBabs:
No thanks, rather stick pins in my eyes

Mail received from:
Imatoyboy4u
Mmm–sexy do you fancy younger men

Reply:
BionicBabs:
No prefer a curry

Fortunately most of the mail I received was complimentary. A lot of it was boring. There was mail from young men living in third world countries who wanted to marry me. I had resentful mail from young girls who thought women of my age shouldn't be on a date site. I promised to forward to them the thousands of mail I had received from young men, strange they didn't reply!
I received mail from women who were worried I might be receiving mail from their men and from men who were worried their women had found out they had sent me mail!!
Then I received mail from *Gemboy*.

GEMBOY:
Hi Babs, my name is Colin. I found your profile captivating, such a pleasure to discover having trawled through the boring, mundane, uninspiring drivel you find on this site. A 54-year-old bubbly extrovert, a renegade in DM's working in a library. Mix that with a touch of bionics and you have an intriguing woman.
I am 56, divorced, not unattractive and have my own PR Company. I live with my two teenage

sons in Bedfordshire, have many interests and enjoy a very active social life, which I share with a large group of friends. I am a whiz in the kitchen and errrm know how to operate the washing machine!! Several of your requirements covered there I hope.

I am happy to talk to you via email until hopefully, you feel comfortable enough to have a chat on the phone?

Here's hoping you reply,

Colin xxx

Colin and I wrote to each other for some time. He was happy to answer all my questions and finally I did feel comfortable enough to give him my phone number.

To me, talking on the phone is really important, you can tell a lot from a voice. Colin was funny, articulate and intelligent and having a really sexy voice didn't count against him. He was a great listener, had the gift of not interrupting when I was on a roll and didn't bore me too much with the details of his failed marriage and never asked for the details of mine.

In the end, again on the spur of the moment, I agreed to meet him and the children had to put up with another 'I don't wanna go' session hours before the rendezvous.

I needn't have worried. Colin and I met at a pub local to me so he had driven a long way. He was patiently waiting in his huge four-wheel drive, not my favourite choice of transport – I need a rope ladder to climb in. I was running my usual half hour late but he still greeted me with a warm hug.

Colin was a member of that nearly extinct breed. He was a true gentleman, in every sense of the word. I loved having the door held open for me. Bob, I recalled, would be on his second pint before I had even struggled through the pub door. Colin helped me off with my jacket and pulled the seat out for me, made sure I was settled, knee tucked away safe from risk of being knocked by any inebriated customers, then went to the bar. I eyed him sneakily whilst his back was turned, not a tall man but nicely put together, immaculately dressed in casual clothing and his presence I noticed demanded attention, as he was served very quickly at the packed bar.

He was easy to talk to, no embarrassing silences when one looks idly around praying for inspiration. We chatted away like old friends. Any interested onlookers would have thought we had known each other for years. This man even lowered the suspension of the four-wheeled drive to make it easier to help me in. Well I think he lowered the suspension, maybe it was magic, I'm no mechanic.

We went for a lovely Chinese meal in a restaurant in Newcastle and he made my night by telling me I had the most beautiful blue eyes. I mean, who couldn't help adoring a man who actually managed to raise his eyes high enough to notice the colour of *your* eyes?

I found myself telling Colin the sad tale of the past few years of my life, leaving out some of the more gory details.

When I finally shut up, appalled that I had revealed so much to this comparative stranger, I looked up and saw such a look of sadness in his lovely kind eyes.

"My God Babs," he said, "You are such a strong woman to have come through all that with two children and still look and sound as cheerful as you do."

"Oh well I'm Bionic," I said, now really horribly embarrassed, kicking myself for exposing so much of my life.

He pulled my arm through his as we walked back to his car. I was grateful as my knee had started to throb painfully and then we drove in silence back to my car where he gave me another hug and we drove away in opposite directions.

"How'd it go?" Lou asked.

"Blew it," I said, shaking my head sadly.

"You going to see him again?" I looked at my daughter, noticing *something* in the intonation of her voice and realised, looking at her troubled face, she wasn't quite ready to share her mother.

"I doubt it," I sighed, "Told him too much about my life."

"What *everything*?" she asked.

"Nearly everything" I nodded.

"Oh my God mother," she laughed, finding a funny side to it.

Just then my mobile rung.

"Babs" – it was Colin, he had allowed enough time for me to get home then pulled over onto the hard shoulder of the M1 to phone me – "I had a lovely time tonight, would really like to see you again if you're OK with that."

"I'd love to," I replied relieved. "I thought I'd blown it, ran off at the mouth too much," I laughed.

"Not at all," he said, "I'm flattered you felt you could tell me. It adds to everything I had already learned about you, a renegade, bubbly extrovert and now I know you are a fighter, altogether it is a very attractive and exciting package," he laughed.

Putting my phone down I noticed the frown had returned to Lou's forehead.

"Come here," I said patting the space next to me on the armchair and as she snuggled against me, the way she had done for so many years I said,

"I'm not going anywhere sweetie, I'm just learning to live again, you have your life and I need mine. Do you understand?"

"Yes," she mumbled, "It just feels so weird."

"To you and me both sweetie," I said. "You and me both."

Over the next few months we became really good friends and slowly but surely, Colin got me to talk about all of my past life. He was wonderful to talk to, sympathetic and wise, constantly offering to be there if I needed him.

My life continued to be like riding a roller coaster, going from enormous highs then plummeting to dark lows. One day, when I was having a particularly bad low, Colin kept phoning me, but I was too upset to speak to him. As I sat weeping at my computer, I noticed him sign in.

"What's up?" he typed. "Talk to me please I'm getting really worried, don't make me drive there to find out what's wrong."

"The bailiffs have paid me a visit," I typed, "Stuck bloody raffle tickets on my furniture, the furniture they are going to take. I'm so tired of the struggle. It just goes on and on."

"Is it the bank?" he asked. Colin knew I owed the bank a lot of money and had put me onto a company that were trying to help me sort things out.

"It's a credit card company, I got it ages ago when I needed just £100 to get my car fixed, I now owe them £700 with all the interest and they want it now."

He put up a little telephone sign and my phone rang, I picked it up.

"Who are they?" he asked. "I'll talk to them, get you time to pay."

"I tried that," I sobbed. "They said it's too late, it's in the hands of the bailiffs."

"Well I'm a Mason," laughed Colin. "Give me the number, I can try, you're too upset to handle this."

"OK, nothing ventured," I sniffed. "Maybe they will listen to you because you're a man," I managed a little laugh.

The next day Colin phoned and said,
"It's sorted."

"You've got me more time?" I asked, excited.

"No, I've paid it," he said simply.

I was shocked, £700, he had paid £700!

"You can't Colin, it will take me forever to pay you back ……"

"Listen," he interrupted, "If you ever find yourself in a position to pay me back then do so but you are not to feel committed to doing it. I admire you tremendously, I like the way you have lead your life, the way you have brought up David and Louise, put yourself through university whilst working. If I have made life just a little bit easier for you by doing this one small thing, then I am happy."

"Colin thank you so much, I just don't know what to say," I almost whispered.

"Then say nothing, we'll chat later, I'll phone you – and take those 'bloody raffle tickets' off your furniture," he laughed and was gone.

"Will you come with me to a ladies' night ball?" Colin asked me one day.

Before I could make my excuses for the usual financial reasons he continued,

"I'll pay for a ball gown and for you to have your hair done and anything else you need, I know money's tight" he teased.

"It will be a nice break for you," he added. You can stay in my spare room over night. I'll cook dinner the next day. What do you say?"

"I'd love to," I said. I really did need something to look forward to, I was relieved he had mentioned the spare room. I adored him but wasn't in love with him and I had recently started to chat to another man, Derek, who I had also met online. I had to admit to myself I was already very attracted to Derek but at this stage, still had no desire to share a bed with anyone.

I'd finally had an arthroscopy on my knee and was feeling less robotic and reckoned I might actually be able to dance by the time the date of the ball came around.

I struggled to find a gown, they were so expensive and half the length needed to be cut away to fit me – such a waste of money for maybe just one wearing.

In the end Colin and I spent a day together going from shop to shop. I was getting hot and bothered trying on so many gowns whilst Colin sat patiently waiting. Then the look on his face told me I'd finally found the right one. He smiled with pleasure when I settled on a lovely black, off the shoulder, fitted, satin gown, decorated simply around the neck with a row of diamante. I already had shoes and a bag that would match. I even had costume jewellery, remnants from the days I used to attend balls with Jim at camp. I was so glad I had a poverty mentality and rarely threw anything away.

Colin looked extremely handsome on the night of the ball in his smart black dinner jacket and trousers with maroon tuxedo and matching bow tie. I so wished I could fall in love with this man and I felt a little tug at my heart when I realised one day I would lose him. One day he would find a woman who would love him the way he so deserved.

I shrugged off the feelings of sadness and went with my Prince Charming to the ball.

It was a truly magical evening, held in the lovely surroundings of Cambridge University. Colin and I danced the night away putting my dodgy knee through every motion and it didn't let me down.

The real test for me was discovering my hosts were Freemasons and not finding myself on the losing side of an argument about secret societies. Being a highly intelligent woman and glancing around at the other guests, I quickly realised I was outnumbered and decided to keep my mouth shut. 'Anyway, they raise a lot of money for charity … and this *was* a free meal.'

Much later, back at Colin's house, dressed in my PJ's – the red ones with little lambs all over them – and lying curled up on my side on one of his wonderfully cosy leather chairs, he stooped down and looking at me said,

"Thanks for being with me, I had a wonderful evening."

"I did too," I said and I think it was at that moment we both knew we would have only a few more lovely evenings together. It was time I gave Colin the chance to move on, to find a woman who would truly love him and make him happy, something at that time I wasn't ready, mentally or physically, to do, if indeed I would ever be.

DEREK

I was still using the chat room, only for fun. I had no interest in dating any men from the site although Tony and I were still firm friends meeting occasionally.

Men who whispered were soon seen off. I just loved to chat in the open room especially when my friends were online. If you can imagine, it's a little bit like being part of a club, sometimes people are there you can chat and joke with, other times the club is full of new-comers and strangers. Or the bullies would be in control, simply talking amongst themselves and intimidating anyone else who tried to join in. There were many of those occasions but if there were enough of us who were not part of their little 'in crowd' we could soon out chat them as if they weren't there and losing power they would leave.

There were persistent whisperers, 'I'm sorry I don't whisper', would only temporarily deter them and they would be back.

It was possible to tell who was popular. As they signed into the room the screen would scroll at a frightening speed as everyone typed a welcome.

It was great being one of those so popular it could take, depending on the speed of your typing, 5 minutes just to say hi back.

As I sat back reading the screen one evening, not at that point in the mood to take part in any of the mundane conversations going on, the screen leapt as *dasman* signed in. I typed in 'hi das' at the end of all the others who had welcomed him and added the little wilted rose now recognised as my signature. Most added smiley faces or thumbs up or a fresh rose and you could use kisses and hearts and several other cute 'emoticons' – little pictures depicting emotions – as you greeted members entering chat.

My little wilted rose had actually been a mistake. I had been looking at the options and spotted it and thinking it looked like my favourite flower, the Snakeshead Frittilery, I started using it, little knowing, but soon discovering, that it actually depicted a wilted flower – but I was stuck with it, and anyway I liked it and no one else was using it.

Within seconds of greeting *dasman* he appeared in my whispers,

"Why the wilted rose Babs?"

"It's not a wilted rose it's a Snakeshead Frittilery and I like it."

"My name is Derek".

"Sorry Derek I don't whisper."

He was gone, only to reappear every time I said hi and even if I didn't say hi but he was one of many so I hardly noticed.

I did notice, however, that he was extremely popular with the ladies, some making fools of themselves trying to get his attention. I also noticed that he loved it and was a total flirt with each and every one of them.

I was desperate at that time to return to Essex. I had never really settled in the Midlands. David and Louise were living with their partners and I was feeling more and more homesick.

Although still working at the library, I was also doing sessional work for the local Youth Offending Team and I loved it. It made sense of my degree and I found I had a natural gift of communication with young people.

This, I decided, was going to be my future – I was going to strive to obtain full time employment with the YOT in Essex. Every time I visited Kate I would call into their office, not only to check on vacancies but also in the hope that they would remember my enthusiasm, and me.

"Where are you Babs?" *Bestgal* asked me in the chat room one day.

BionicBabs: In the Midlands Bestie but I'm an Essex girl and I wanna go home (here I added a little weeping emoticon)

Bestgal: awwwwwww Babs can't you go home then

BionicBabs: I need a job Bestie, I want to work with naughty young people

I noticed my whisper light flashing and was determined to get rid of the intruder. *Bestgal* and I often had fun in the chat room and I wanted to get to main room chatting.

"Hi Babs, Derek, remember me?"
"Yes," I replied. "The chat room flirt and I still don't whisper!"

"Hold on, I just wanted to tell you I work for a young peoples' drug and alcohol service, maybe I can help you."

This immediately got my attention and we started to talk about work with young people. Derek suggested we went onto messenger and I agreed it was less complicated on there, at least you could see when the other person was typing making a written conversation flow.

He was charming, attractive, intelligent and in a caring profession. His profile stated he was separated from his wife and I was warmed when he told me he saw his three children every weekend and they came first, way before any woman he might meet. Of course I could completely identify with that, having dedicated the last 10 years of my life exclusively to my children.

He told me he had been a musician in the Guards, had travelled widely and worked abroad, always with young people. All this information he backed up with photographs and it didn't escape me that Derek had always been an exceptionally attractive man. I felt comfortable talking to him, looked forward to our conversations and at some point we started flirting with each other.

It was quite innocent to start with. Derek asked me about the men in my life since my divorce and was staggered when I told him I had been celibate for 10 years and had only recently started dating.

"What no one?" he typed.

"No one."

"No sex?"

"No sex."

"My God, how did you manage?"

"Easy," I replied, "My children were most important, I was studying and working all hours, I had a social life as such, I just put everything else on hold."

"I couldn't do that," Derek wrote, "I need sex."

"Well that's men for you," I replied, "And you have your wife looking after your children. I would never have taken a man home and certainly couldn't see myself in some seedy hotel room so I just didn't think about it and was happy with my decision."

"So if I take you to bed, it will be like having a virgin."

"A born again virgin," I replied, adding an emoticon with a huge grin on its face.

BORN AGAIN VIRGIN

Derek went away for a week with his eldest son. He emailed me most days and sent photographs of them together in frozen Poland. When he returned home – without too much persuasion from him – I finally gave him my phone number.

He phoned me the very next morning, waking me from a deep sleep.
"Who is this?" I mumbled.
He laughed,
"I don't know, she gives me her phone number one day and doesn't know who it is the next."
"Derek?" I asked now fully awake.
"Yes" he laughed.
"Ooooh nice voice," I said, curling up in my cosy bed with the phone tucked under my ear.
"Where are you?" he asked, "You sound muffled."
"In bed," I laughed, "You woke me up."
"Well stay there, I'll be with you in four hours."
"Put your foot down," I replied.

Derek started to phone me every day, two or three times a day – driving to work, driving from work and between appointments.
It was just before my knee operation and I had been seeing Colin for some time. They knew about each other, Colin accepting reluctantly that our relationship wasn't exclusive and Derek occasionally making sarcastic comments about 'Bedford man.'

The day came when Derek phoned me and said, "I have Friday off can I come and see you?"

My heart did a flick flack across the room … did I really want this and how could I meet this man when I was still crippled? His profile said he was 6' I'm 5'1", had he really taken on board I was a midget? Did I look like my photos? Hell no my hair was 6" longer! Did that matter? Should I tell him, or should I just make an excuse – like my other knee's just broken, or maybe both my arms?!!

"OK," I said weakly.

So it was arranged, he was going to visit me in four days' time. God I felt sick.

The fear I had over meeting Tony and Colin came nowhere close to the fear I was now feeling. I could honestly say I had liked both of them but with Derek I knew I was already feeling 'chemistry,' even though we hadn't actually met.

My confidence plummeted. I even discussed it with Colin who told me somewhat sadly, that he knew 'what's-his-name' would be bowled over by me.

The day came. Derek was due to arrive at 10.00 and my hair was still sopping wet.

Right on the dot of 10.00 my mobile rung.

"I'm in Madeley, where are you?"

I told him I wasn't ready and begged him to kill about 15 minutes.

"I'll try," he said, sounding reluctant but I have been driving non-stop since 7 o'clock this morning and I need the loo."

Ten minutes later he phoned again,

"That's it I need the loo desperately now."

"OK, OK," and I gave him the directions. He was only two minutes away from my house and oh well, my troublesome hair was still sopping but at least I had make-up on.

This giant of a man stooped to peck me on the cheek as I held the door open for him then dashing up stairs he cried,

"Where's the bloody toilet?"

Hmm, *not* a good start.

A few minutes later and probably very relieved, he joined me in the kitchen and as I glanced around at him I thought I caught a look of disappointed resignation on his handsome face.

Derek had long curly white hair and a 'goatee.' He had lovely dark brown eyes but there was detachment in them.

'Oh dear,' I thought, what a disappointment, 'I'm so not going to like you *dasman*'!!

Yes he was tall and very handsome and I loved the way he was dressed, blue jeans and matching denim shirt and tan boots.

We sat down and chatted and actually got on quite well but the conversation was often about him and mostly about the tall, beautiful young blonde women he had dated, even telling me his wife used to be a model.

I really wasn't that bothered, thinking,

'Well you lucked out this time Mr. Tough Luck.'

Although I had reluctantly cooked a curry for dinner I had not prepared anything for lunch so Derek suggested we drove to a local pub.

He also had a four-wheel drive but so unlike Colin, I had to clamber into the dam thing, gammy knee and all, without any help.

On the way to the pub, he told me he went home every weekend and I thought, 'yes you have already told me that'.

He also pointed out that he had no intention of getting a divorce for at least another two years, not until his children were independent.

Again I wasn't bothered. I was rapidly losing interest in this man.

I was two minutes behind him entering the pub, nearly being hit in the face by the door after he had pushed through it. He found himself a nice comfortable seat at a table and picked up the menu whilst I struggled to sit comfortably, protecting my knee. That was a point to remember … he hadn't even asked me how it was or how I was feeling although he knew I was having an operation in a weeks' time.

The scampi and chips were lovely but the conversation, yet again, returned to him. This was a man comfortable and used to talking about himself and I resigned myself to putting up with the rest of the day as best I could.

Dinner at home was far better. Lou joined us and I have to admit he was excellent with her. I could understand why he was so successful working with children. I had no appetite and busied myself in the kitchen whilst they tucked into curried chicken, chatting away like old friends.

After the meal, when Louise had gone to meet friends, he fell asleep on the sofa and I went onto the computer to have some friendly, fun conversation in the chat room.

A couple of my friends – of my envious friends – knew he was meeting me today,

Bestgal: has he gone
BionicBabs: no he's asleep on the sofa
wilma: what you done to him
BionicBabs: nothing, he's all warn out talking about himself
Bestgal: is he as gorgeous as he looks in his pics
BionicBabs: Yep, wannim? He's gonna be back on the market lol

Derek woke up and I quickly shut down the computer.
"I'd better go," he said wearily, "I'm going to stay the night with my mother."
"OK," I said, smiling.
At the door I thanked him for a nice day.
"It's been really nice meeting you but it won't be repeated," I said and happily noted he was genuinely surprised.
"Oh, that bad?" he asked puzzled.
"Not great," I laughed, maybe a little too heartily.
I felt relieved as he pulled out of the drive 'and that' I thought 'was that.'

It wasn't! To my amazement he phoned me the very next morning as if the day before had been a complete success, not the total disaster I remembered.

He was happy, jovial and chatty, talking about the next time we would meet and what we would do.

He was so much nicer to talk to on the phone, when you couldn't see the lack of emotion in his eyes or the disappointment on his face.

I soon realised Derek was not used to failure and that rejection just made the quarry more exciting.

I was naïve however and apt to dismiss such small failures in a life that was so packed with massive disasters. Once more I became swept along by his new found enthusiasm and looked forward to his phone calls and seeing him online in the chat room.

The chat room for us was a disaster. Derek was an incorrigible flirt, lapping up all the attention he got from the ladies and there was plenty of that. What surprised me was how jealous he could become when I was on the receiving end of attention from men and there was plenty of that too.

On one occasion, when I was joking with several men he exited the chat room returning about 30 minutes later and taking up his flirting with renewed zeal.

One thing that should have concerned me and certainly would now, was Derek's insistence that we kept our relationship quiet from others in chat. His reason? He felt jealousy would make some of them very nasty. 'Some', I thought, 'were pretty nasty already,' but I agreed to go along with it, omitting to tell him that a few already knew.

But 'keeping our relationship quiet' didn't stop him making references to his trip to the Midlands and several references to my house, or giving me a special welcome when I signed into the chat room. I found the whole arrangement, in fact the relationship, very, very confusing but hung in there, still believing there was something special happening between us.

I finally went into hospital to have the long awaited operation on my knee. Reluctantly the doctors let me go home the same day, mainly because I begged and when refused, started humming the tune to *The Great Escape* and encouraging other post op patients to give me a 'leg up' so I could escape out of the window.

Colin sent a card and flowers. Tony phoned to wish me well. Derek? Well nothing from Derek.

I spent hours watching television and reading for a second time my favourite Stephen King book, 'Needful Things,' which gave me an idea – I could probably sit at my computer using my needlework box as a footstool with which to prop up my still painful knee.

It worked a treat and I signed into 50's chat room. Most of the chatters knew I had been in hospital and surprised to see me so soon were asking how I was.

I noticed *dasman* was on what I called 'the guest list' but was not taking part in the room conversation, then suddenly ...

Beautifulblonde05: thanks das nice chatting, I'll let you know (followed by several big red kisses and a heart)
Dasman: you're welcome darling I'll be waiting

My friend Julie (*Wilma*) joined the conversation,

dasman: hello Wilma xx
BionicBabs: wilms hi mate
Dasman: hello Babs xx
BionicBabs: hi das xx
Wilma: Babbbbbbbbbbbbbbbbs hi what you doin home thought you'd be in for a few days????
BionicBabs: other patients helped me escape wilms lol

I had been ignoring my flashing 'whisper' lights for sometime but noticed Derek, in his guise as *dasman*, had joined the queue. I clicked on his name.
"Hi Babs, why haven't you been answering your mobile?" "They don't let you answer your phone when you're on the operating table."
"Oh your operation, how did it go?"
"I'll never play the piano again, gotta go, see ya". And with that I clicked out of the room.
I sat back in my chair, confused and upset. My knee was throbbing. In the lounge I could hear my mobile ringing. I ignored it, I knew it would be Derek and I wanted to get my head together before I spoke to him. I was hurt and I didn't like

the feeling. I wasn't used to it. Yes Bob had hurt me physically and mentally but somehow that was different, he was a slave to alcohol. Other than that the last time I had been hurt was by Ken when I was in my early 20's. I had learned a lot from that experience and vowed never to let it happen again.

I thought, now in my 50's, I was safe from that type of pain but well Derek, how could he forget my operation and then be so nonchalant about it? I didn't give *beautifulblonde05* a thought at that time but weeks later, I would. I had so much to learn.

Within a couple of days, Derek and I were 'back to normal' – whatever that is. He was phoning again regularly and we chatted for hours online. We planned to meet again two weeks after the ball and although I knew Colin and I were coming to a close I was excited about my relationship with Derek. He often made reference to my second virginity and how he wanted to be the one to take it and I knew I was hoping for the same.

Two weeks after the ball with Colin, Derek came to see me again and this time we didn't even wait for the kettle to boil. We went straight upstairs to my bedroom and I happily gave up my second virginity. I knew instantly, that Derek wasn't making love to me. This was sex, nothing more, special to me but, I knew, not special to him.

I was totally hooked on him, the first man I had taken to my bed in 10 years and that was very special to me. Looking back, I know I didn't love him but that was because there was always this invisible barrier, a barrier he would bring slamming down whenever he felt I was getting too close to him.

Later, whilst we were driving to have something to eat, Derek said,

"I'm happy for us to continue like this, just let me know if you want to go with someone else and I'll let you know."

I didn't really understand what he meant 'go with someone else,' did he think I would sleep with several different men at once? I hadn't when I was young, I certainly wasn't going to start at 54.

"The weekends are out," he continued, "I spend those with the family and the children will always come first."

"Hold on," I said putting my hands up to stop him, "Are you saying you spend every weekend at home with your wife and children?"

"Yes," said Derek, "I go home on Friday evening, I have my own room there and I stay there until Sunday or Monday morning. There's no sex, my wife doesn't want it anymore but she's the mother of my children and I respect and value her for that."

I was struggling to get my head around this. He still lived with his family at the weekends. I was just wanted for sex. Was that what he was saying?

Why didn't I finish with him there and then? Well I had just given myself to him, my first sex in 10 years. It simply *had* to mean something more.

Of course it didn't. Derek was what I now call a 'chat room predator'. He would seek out vulnerable, or better still willing women, who would satisfy him sexually with absolutely no strings attached.

This was not, however, my nature. Apart from the occasional platonic date, I dedicated myself to Derek for four long years, even though I knew he was sleeping with many, many other women.

It was four years of pain and humiliation.

In the chat room he continued to flirt with any and every woman, probably even worse than before. On one occasion, one woman who often liked to share things with me 'whispered' and asked me to look at her new boyfriend and then named *dasman*. This particular woman had a very poor reputation in chat, she was well known for sending men naked photographs of herself in different obscene poses. When I mentioned this to Derek, he admitted he had received several but had deleted them because they were so dreadful. I wondered what he would have done had it been a more 'attractive' woman. Many chatters realised there was 'something' between us and I started to receive nasty emails. Some accused me of taking Derek from them. Some said they were seeing him regularly. I was told he 'whispered' many women and always denied knowing me if challenged.

Then *beautifulblonde05* emailed me. She told me she had had an 8-month relationship with Derek and recently he had been pestering her to renew it. The sad thing was, I believed her.

I still remained faithful to him although I rarely saw him. On the few occasions I did back off he intensified his attention. The signals were so confusing I really didn't know what to think.

On the one hand there was this dreadful chat room tart of a man and on the other an intelligent, sweet, caring Derek who went out of his way to help me fulfil my dream of returning to Essex. He suggested careers with young people, suggested *Connextions* and when I applied for a job with the Youth Offending Service, he not only gave me a reference but he also persuaded his local YOT drug and alcohol worker to phone me the morning of the interview to give me some good advice on things to say and likely questions I would be asked.

I was offered the job and Derek was the first person I phoned to tell. He sounded genuinely pleased for me.

"Love you," he said.

"Yeh right," I said, disbelievingly.

The relationship continued in this manner, even when I moved back to Essex. I occasionally saw him and occasionally spoke to him on the phone. He never ever put himself out for me and he continued to flirt in the chat room as if I didn't exist.

He confused me even more when my old car started to give me real problems. I had to have a car for work and Derek phoned me, told me he wanted to get another car as he was finding his little Mazda too small.

"Do you want the Mazda?" he asked, "I'm happy for you to pay when you can, it's a great little car, you won't have problems with it."

Such thoughtfulness just added to my confusion but I accepted, relieved I was at last going to have a reliable car and a pretty red one at that. Days later, he broke my heart.

I was dreadfully lost, had been driving in circles for hours and was getting very tired. I phoned Derek and he talked me through to the right direction and road and then stayed on the phone and chatted to me as I drove home.

"Been with anyone else since you met me?" I joked.

"Errrm yes," he replied. "The other night, bumped into an old girlfriend. We went for a meal. We were both lonely, horny, needy and so we had sex. What about you, you been with anyone?"

"No," was all I could say. I was devastated, unable to speak I switched off my phone and drove the next 25 miles in tears.

I stayed faithful to Derek for another two years but we only had sex twice in that time.

He started to have little digs at me – my age, looks, height and I put up with it all until he came back from a two-week holiday in the States.

"Did you spend any time with women?" I asked him online one night.

"Yes," he wrote, "spent a few days with one then a week in a hotel with another."

I asked him how he could do that, spend so much time with women he hardly knew when he could only give me at the most the occasional weekend.

"I needed somewhere to stay," he wrote.

He told me the second one was only 36 and she cried when he left but he couldn't understand it she knew 'what's what' he wrote. I found myself feeling sorry for this young woman, if she felt half the pain I had felt and indeed was feeling then she was really suffering.

This however was my wake up call. Derek had changed beyond all recognition. He had used chat rooms for years and was now using dating sites. I have no idea why he continued with me for such a long time. I hate to say it but maybe it was because I was so convenient and so stupid.

I think, online, it's just far too easy for a good-looking man with a good job and a plausible reason for staying married to 'pull' if you like, vulnerable women.

I have to thank Derek for finally making me grow up. Can I still be used? Absolutely not! Now I ask many questions. I don't date men who are married, separated or 'in an open' relationship. I don't date men who have been online for more than six months without a damn good reason. Any longer and they are already hooked on internet dating and trawling through the endless photographs of women. And I don't date men from chat rooms – in fact I rarely use them. I stick to one dating site because it tells me everything I

need to know and there is a bond between the women who share information about 'predators.'
I still occasionally speak to Derek online. He hasn't changed and I think he accepts that he is now too selfish to want to change. He is still married and still has many partners. He would hate it if he knew how sorry I feel for him.
I feel sorry for him because I think he's lonely.
I feel sorry for him because I think the only time he doesn't feel lonely is when he is in bed with some woman or has that to look forward to.
I feel sorry for him … because he lost me.

DAVID

I was on my way home and was so excited that I was tempted to put my foot down and do a ton up down the motorway. I swear the air felt warmer as I crossed from Cambridgeshire into Essex ... nearly there now.

I'd got my dream: Final Warnings Project Worker for the Youth Offending Team. What a change that environment was going to be after six years in a university library working with some of the most promising and privileged young people.
I loved Keele and was sad to leave. I'd made some really good friends who stood by me when things got tough and the worse thing was, I was leaving my beloved children behind. Louise was now working for Camp America in the United States, having been encouraged by Derek, who'd worked for them in the past.
David was living with his girlfriend and her little girl and had taken the Midlands to his heart, having even lost his Essex accent. I doubted he would ever return home and I knew how desperately I was going to miss my son who had so often been my right hand.

I recalled a time in Braintree when I had been totally handicapped by a trapped nerve in my neck, in agony most of the time and drugged to the hilt. David, at the tender age of 11, had been forced to look after Lou in the mornings, making sure she'd had breakfast and was dressed ready for school, then walking with her whilst I watched concerned from Lou's bedroom window. I knew at the bottom of the road Jayne would be there to meet them and see them safely across the road and into school, but I hated watching them go on their own.

I was totally helpless. Kate came as often as she could but there came a day when, desperate for some shopping to be done, I wrote a list for David and then watched him walk until out of sight, the 200 yards to the nearest supermarket.

I kept watch for what seemed like hours. It was pouring with rain when I suddenly spotted him walking back, no shopping in his hands.

I managed to crawl downstairs and was waiting when he struggled through the backdoor and almost fell into the kitchen, his hair and clothes dripping wet, eyes glistening and cheeks bright red from the wet and cold.

"Where's Lou?" he asked, "I need help."

Lou came downstairs and David told her to empty his hood and his pockets whilst he removed the shopping he'd pushed up his sleeves and zipped up inside his jacket.

It's hard to explain the pain I felt when he explained that the shopping bags had burst spilling the goods all over the path. Although David smiled happily, telling me how people had stopped to help, stuffing things into every part of his clothing, I felt dreadful imagining the distress he probably hadn't felt.

"I was fine mum," he said, noticing my worried face and trying to reassure me, "I'll go again when we need stuff."

"I'll go too," said Louise.

"*Oh no you won't,*" David and I had said in unison, laughing as Louise put her hands on her hips and stomped back to her bedroom.

Moving to the Midlands hadn't come too soon for David. Just a few months before we left, he had been attacked one morning whilst on his way to catch the school bus. He was just 13, tiny for his age and reaching out for that independency we mothers are so afraid and reluctant to give them. I had been driving him to the bus station every morning but finally, more for convenience sake, because Lou had to be taken in the opposite direction, I said he could walk the 10-minute journey on his own.

Within one week he was attacked, it is thought, by someone sleeping rough, who had grabbed him from behind, knocked him out, took his Walkman and left him unconscious.

The man was never found but David's smashed Walkman was – it had probably been broken in the struggle. David became afraid to go out, even into the garden, on his own. He was nervous whenever someone was walking behind him.

Once in the Midlands, David returned to his old self, happily going off on his bike to play with his newfound friends.

YOU DON'T KNOW WHAT IT'S LIKE

I had never been so far away from my children and with each mile I tucked behind me my heart filled with a sense of loss that threatened to overwhelm me.

I pulled into a service, opened the sunroof of my car, laid back and stared at the beautiful clear blue sky.

I would love to say I had been a super mum, protecting my children from all ill whilst they followed me along the rocky road of my life. I would love to say they had come away unscathed and were perfectly rounded healthy young adults. I would dearly love to say all this, but I can't.
Both my children have suffered and I would warn any parent whose life has been similar to mine who, even though their children have shared such suffering, still say 'there's nothing wrong with my kids – hasn't affected them at all'. Well *watch this space*! It may not be evident now, but it may well be later on in life.

My sweet son, although constantly saying, 'I'm nothing like dad,' seemed hell bent on proving Jeffrey Helm wrong, who wrote:

'The genetics of alcoholism mirrors what has become increasingly apparent to geneticists: life is complicated. The way you act or many genes interacting with each other along with various environmental factors likely influence the quality of your health. The concept that a small number of

genes are responsible for disease or behaviour is obsolete. What that means, in the case of alcoholics or drug addicts, is that even if your parents were addicted, it's unlikely that their genes are the deciding factor that will make you an addict.'
(Jeffrey Helm, July 2006: http://thetyee.ca/News/2006/07/28/AddictGene/).

I remembered an occasion when David had angrily sworn he would never be like his father.
They had been so excited. Louise was to be a bridesmaid for the first time at the wedding of Chris and Gemma, a young man and his fiancé with whom Bob shared a house. They had often found themselves looking after the children when their father had had them for the weekend and simply disappeared.
David and Louise adored them. They treated the children with more consideration and gave them more love than their father would have done, or ever did or could. The children would come home full of tales of their weekend and the fun things they had done, Louise often with biscuits and cakes she had cooked with Gemma.
Sadly, I had only met them on a couple of occasions when picking the children up, but I always knew it was *they* who had shared the responsibility for the children that weekend. David and Louise would be smiling happily, they would be clean, as would their clothes, all neatly packed into their little cases.

Although they didn't really know me they still invited me to the wedding. Sadly I had to refuse but promised to be at the church. I knew I couldn't be in the same room as Bob, especially when there was alcohol around.

Louise looked beautiful, her thick black hair tied up in ringlets. Her dress, hand made by the bride's mother, was Little-Bo-Peep style, in rich cream and deep red brocade and she wore little matching cream ballet shoes. She carefully carried a basket of flowers.

David was handsome and very grown up in his first suit. He was so looking forward to spending time with his dad.

"He'll have to be smart, won't he mum?" he'd asked, more used to seeing his father scruffy and hung over.

I knew instantly at the church that Bob was terribly hung over. His eyes were red, his speech slurred and his hands were shaking uncontrollably.

I think the bride's mother could see the concern in my eyes as I hung onto the hands of my children.

"Don't worry, we'll take very good care of them," she smiled cocking her head toward her husband and family standing close by.

I drove away but spent the rest of the day watching the clock leaving an hour early to pick them up.

The beautiful bride greeted me warmly giving me a plate of food she had carefully saved for me.

"David sat with us on the top table," she said, "And Louise was wonderful".

As I looked nervously around the hall for my former husband, I smiled when I spotted Louise running around with other children. David was dancing with his aunty Jean. Bob had four older sisters, Jean being the eldest and a younger brother Jack, an usher with Bob at the wedding. Jack nodded to me from the other side of the room but made no attempt to come over and say hi.

'Strange', I thought, I usually got on so well with the other members of Bob's family.

Jean came over with David who immediately wrapped his arms tightly around my waste.

"Where's Bob?" I asked her, still nervously looking around.

"I don't know," she replied, "I'll see you later," and with that she walked away.

I looked down at my son still holding onto me as if I would disappear had he relinquished his hold.

"Where's daddy?" I asked him.

"I don't know," he said looking up at me, his eyes, close to tears, were full of sorrow.

"Please can we go?" he begged.

We collected the now weary Louise, said our goodbyes and walked out to the car. David scrambled into the seat next to me and Louise I noticed, glancing into my rear view mirror, was asleep before we had even left the village hall car park.

"How was it?" I asked David.

"OK" he said softly.

"Where was daddy?" David's response to this question knocked me sick. He sobbed hysterically, struggling for breath.

"I don't know," he managed to say, "After the church he said … he said … daddy said he had to get something and he left and he didn't ever come back," he sobbed.

I pulled over and turned the engine off, gathering my heartbroken son into my arms.

"I was on my own," he cried, "Till Gemma came for me and put me next to Lou, I was on my own. I'll *never* be like him, never, never, never!"

I held onto him tightly as he cried out the pain, feeling every sob rip through his small body.

When he finally fell asleep, occasionally whimpering, I laid him back in his seat, checked his safety belt and carefully pulled away and drove home.

I decided this had to stop. Bob could not be allowed to hurt my children any longer and it was at that moment that I decided to accept Keele's offer of a place on their graduate course.

David started to drink alcohol at the age of 16, he left home at 17 and by 18 he was addicted. He drifted from job to job and try as I might to stay in touch, there were long periods when I didn't know where he was or how he was.

Years later, when he had settled down with Kim and made me a grandma for the fist time to little Ellie, he told me he'd left home because he was already fighting his addiction to alcohol. He'd hated himself and hadn't wanted to put me through what I'd suffered with his father.

My dear son hadn't changed. He was still the caring, loving and thoughtful son he'd always been. I hadn't done *so* badly.

YOU DON'T KNOW WHAT IT'S LIKE

LOUISE

As I lay with my face toward the sun in that noisy services car park, no longer in a rush to get to Essex, my thoughts drifted to my daughter Louise, so far away in America – how I missed her. David and I had driven her to Heathrow to see her off. I had dreaded it as Bob had decided to be there too.

I needn't have worried. He looked old and frail, shorter even. 'Try to hit me now,' I thought, feeling brave with my tall son beside me, a protective arm around my shoulders.

Lou looked so young as she waved happily goodbye, her long hair in plaits, a cap, as always on her head, huge rucksack over her shoulders.

I finally let the tears flow as she disappeared from view. David held up one strong arm toward his father, who had made a move to comfort me. Instead David wrapped his arms around me.

"Don't cry mum, it will be good for her, maybe she will stop … well you know what."

Yes, I knew what he meant and quietly I was praying for the same thing.

I recalled a day some years back, when David and Lou had walked into the lounge hand in hand and David had said,

"Show mummy Lou," pushing her hair back from her face.

"Do you think there's something wrong with me mum?" Louise asked.

At first I didn't know exactly what I was looking at and then I realised … she had no hair from the top of her temple, back about 2 inches and down to just behind her ears. Her scalp was as smooth as a baby's bottom, there was no sign of growth at all.

My hands flew to my mouth my eyes staring, I couldn't take in what I was seeing. Lou wore her hair in a bob combed forward therefore hiding this loss of hair.

"She pulls it out mummy, I've seen her do it," David told me.

"WHY Lou, why do you do it?" I asked.

"Because it releases endorphins," she said, practically, apparently unconcerned and smiling.

She was just 12 years old and here she was telling me quite calmly, she pulled her hair out by the roots because it released endorphins.

I knew it released endorphins, I'd got a bloody psychology degree, and then it hit me, she had looked up Self Harming in my psychology books and found an answer she could run with.

Louise had developed a condition called Trichotillomania, a compulsive behaviour. People with Trichotillomania pull hair out at the root from places like the scalp, eyebrows and eyelashes. Some people pull large handfuls of hair, which can leave bald patches on the scalp or eyebrows. Lou would pull out her hair one strand at a time. She would inspect the strand after pulling it out and play with it. She often put the hair in her mouth, nibbled off the root and discarded the hair.

YOU DON'T KNOW WHAT IT'S LIKE

This activity and other forms of self-harm, and this is what Lou was doing, she was self-harming, is thought to release endorphins. Endorphins interact with opiate receptor neurons to reduce the intensity of pain.

Besides behaving as a pain regulator, endorphins are also thought to be connected to physiological processes including euphoric feelings, appetite modulation and the release of sex hormones.

In a nutshell, Lou was not only feeling no pain when she pulled out her hair because of the endorphins, but she was also getting a kick from it. The psychologist in me instantly recognised there must be something very wrong with my little girl if she needed this endorphin rush so much she was prepared to pull her hair out to achieve it. However, the mother in me reacted appallingly.

"You have to stop Lou," I almost shouted, a mixture of shock and fear in my voice.

"How?" she asked innocently, "I've been trying to." Idiotically I said,

"Just stop for God's sake!"

"I can't," she said, beginning to get upset, "can't you stop me?" I grabbed her to me and rocked her on my lap whilst I attempted to quell my own panic. 'This won't kill her' I thought, 'its not anorexia or bulimia, she's not cutting herself or swallowing stuff.'

More panic surged, I felt her body ... no she wasn't starving. I pulled up her sleeves examining her arms and then her legs ... no sign of cuts new or old. I resisted asking her whether she ever

229

swallowed anything harmful, she looked, apart from her hair, far too healthy. 'No, she's not killing herself, we can get through this.'

David squeezed next to us on the armchair,

"I should have told you before mum but I didn't know how bad it was," he said, sadly shaking his head.

"Not your fault," said Lou, stroking his own healthy head of hair, tears now pouring down her face.

"I *can* stop can't I mum, now that you know, I can stop?"

"Yes darling," I answered though my mind was screaming 'but how?'

I didn't sleep that night I was overridden with feelings of self-loathing and guilt. It was the way I had led my life that was causing my children to suffer. It was *my* fault. What was the use of a psychology degree if I couldn't pick up on things, if I couldn't help *them*?

I thought I had always encouraged my children to talk to me, they could tell me anything and I think to a large degree they did, but I also recognised they had this desire to protect me, not to upset me – they had lived with my pain and didn't want to add to it or be a cause of more.

I could recall times when they would say, 'I don't want to upset you but ...' or 'don't get upset mum but ...' but never 'don't get angry'. My anger, it occurred to me, was acceptable to them, my pain wasn't.

I realised now, maybe too late, that they needed to know they *could* upset me and I would get over it.

Being upset was part of life and would be fleeting and in the aftermath things would get sorted and life would go on with no great damage done.

How much more didn't I know about my own children? What other important parts of their lives were hidden from me?

I got out of bed and went into Lou's room. She was fast asleep, her hair had slipped to one side and I could see in the moonlight the huge bald patch on her tiny head. 'Why was she doing this, there had to be a reason?' I thought.

She was doing so well, a high achiever she had passed her 11+ and was in her first year at Newcastle-under-Lyme's best school, a fee paying school but Lou had got a place on scholarship.

I was aware she didn't have many friends. She had always been outspoken and far too advanced for her years, even occasionally intimidating teachers.

I could remember one occasion when she was at junior school in Essex, her class teacher was not selecting her for anything. Lou had always had starring parts in school plays. On one occasion, in her first infant year, she had been the narrator, standing on her own and reading from a book into a microphone whilst others acted out the scenes.

"She's very advanced," Mr McDonnell, now her headmaster as well as David's, had said.

She also took part in other activities like dancing and sport but suddenly she was the back end of an animal or sitting on a bench whilst others performed. She was part of a dancing display, I recalled, and so was the rest of the class, but Lou was wearing a hastily found adult skirt, hurriedly pinned to make it fit. She spent the whole routine tugging at the skirt to keep it up. I also noticed, she was dancing with a girl and not a boy but swept that aside, 'it's a dirty job but someone has to do it,' I thought.

Concerned, I went to see her class teacher, maybe Lou was being punished for some misdemeanour or the other.

I had always got on with Miss Edwards, she had gone to Keele and I was due to start there at the beginning of the new semester.

There was something about the way she was talking about Lou that caused me to raise my hands to stop her and interrupt with,

"Can I ask you, do you like my daughter?"

"No," she replied caught off guard, "You should teach her how to be a little girl. I'm sick to death of her always correcting me – my spelling – and then the other day for getting the year of the Battle of Hastings wrong. I said 1086, slip of the tongue, that was the War of the Roses, I meant 1066.

I stood up slowly and leant across her desk my furious face inches from her smug one,

"*You're* a teacher – how dare you tell me what I should teach my daughter to be. You madam, are in the wrong profession, you should accept every child for who they are."

I turned back to her as I left her classroom and added,

"Oh and by the way, 1086 was the year the Domesday Book was completed, 1089 was the year of the War of the Roses and 1066 was indeed the Battle of Hastings. I suggest you do your homework before you start dishing it out!!"

I stormed into Mr McDonnell's office – who for once was supportive. He was outraged when I repeated my conversation with Miss Edwards.

"I will sort this Mrs Cunningham, this is not the behaviour I expect from my teachers. If it's any comfort, I have always thought how refreshing Louise is – how bright and intelligent, such a mature head on such young shoulders. Mrs Edwards is leaving at the end of the year, until then I suggest Louise go into the year above, I am certain she will cope."

Louise went into a higher year and certainly did cope especially as she was so much happier.

Even then, she hadn't told me what was happening at school and it hurt me to think she had been in that wretched woman's class for 8 months without complaining.

Recalling this, I wondered if school was having an affect on Louise and determined to talk to her as soon as possible.

The next day at breakfast I asked casually,

"How's school going Lou?"

"OK," she replied not looking up.

I knew – instantly I knew – nothing was ever 'OK' to my daughter, the queen of exaggeration and performance. Things were, 'fabulous darling', 'fantastic', 'superb' or the opposite, 'absolutely dreadful', 'appalling', 'horrendous'.

With a knowing look, David mentioned something about bike and friends and tactfully left the room.

I sat opposite Lou and asked gently, taking her small hand in mine,

"What's up with school Louise?"

At first she didn't answer, just continued to stare at her empty serial bowl. Then she looked at me,

"What makes you think there's anything wrong?" she asked, lowering her eyes once again.

"Look at me Lou," I said and looking into her eyes, "I know because OK is not part of your usual vocabulary. If you are now using OK it means something is not OK … OK?"

She laughed.

"It's a good school mum, you were so proud when I got in."

"I was *very* proud Lou, proud of your achievement but it only has a reputation of being good academically. If you aren't happy there you must tell me, talk to me please."

"I hate it," she burst out. "Do you know on our first day we were asked to put our hands up if we had a swimming pool and then tennis courts, boats and what cars and a home gym, never even heard of one of those. Then it was 'what does your father do for a living?' The girls are nasty, they hate me, make fun of my trainers and sports bag and everything. I'm on my own all the time. Then when Dawn's mum started to give me a lift, Dawn told everyone what a horrid scruffy little house I lived in."

Now the floodgates were open she was unable to stop …

"Then the other day, we were kept in at lunch time 'cos it was pouring and they let me play blind man's bluff – mum I was so pleased, it was the first time they let me join in anything. They blindfolded me, spun me around and then shoved me out in the rain. I was soaked through to my skin, got sent home, got told off first, then sent home."

I remembered a day Louise had come home cold and soaking wet, claiming she had lost her bus fare and walked three miles home.

"Was that the day?" I asked. Lou nodded.

"Did you lose your money and walk home?"

"No. Well I didn't lose my money but I walked home to stretch time out."

"Why didn't you phone me Lou, you had enough money to phone, I would have picked you up?"

"Mum, I didn't want you to know, I didn't want you to worry."

There it was *she didn't want me to worry*. This had to stop.

"It's my job to worry, it's part of being a mother. I can't bear to think you've been going through this for what, 8 months? Don't you realise this is bullying?"

Lou laughed at that.

"Don't you know there is no bullying at my school? I told them once I had been punched in the stomach by one of the girls when I was on my way to the bus station and they just pushed it aside and told me to take another route."

I was truly shocked, horrified that anyone could have been violent towards my child but, try as I might, she would not give me the name of the girl who had hit her.

I was furious, what an outrageous way for any school to behave and surely the teacher who asked them about swimming pools and tennis courts must have known there were children there from far poorer backgrounds. Yes this school had mostly extremely wealthy, fee-paying children but it also had children like Louise who had *earned* their place and had a right to be there.

I telephoned the school the following Monday and demanded to see the head teacher and after a pause was told I could see him at 2 pm sharp that afternoon.

Although I had seen the school many times before, it now looked very intimidating. The huge red brick buildings with its stained glass and leaded windows surrounded by acres of green playing fields, had a long and distinguished history, some said it had been traced back over four hundred years. It was said to have been modelled on Dr Arnold's Rugby School.

I imagined how nervous Louise must have felt on her first days here, coming from a small village school to this daunting place.

I parked my battered old car behind a Rolls Royce and hoped to God I wouldn't have to take a hammer to the engine to get it going when I left.

Like a naughty girl I sat waiting outside the headmaster's office, horribly aware that coming straight from university had meant I wasn't exactly power dressed – nope, old blanket coat, Keele scarf, leggings tucked into slouch socks and Doc Martens wasn't exactly power dressing.

Walking into the office I was immediately aware that I was out-numbered and probably out-manoeuvred. Sitting – I am sure with plenty of legroom – behind his huge mahogany desk was the headmaster, the girls' head teacher, the year teacher and Louise's kindly class teacher, Mrs Allan, the only one who looked at me with sympathy.

"Mob-handed I see," I said, as ever saying the first thing that popped into my head.

"Not at all Ms Cunningham," hissed the headmaster pointing to a seat in front of his desk.

Not wishing to shout, I moved the chair about a foot closer to the panel of teachers.

"How can we help you?" he asked, a smile on his lips that failed to reach his eyes.

"My daughter is being bullied," I replied.

"We don't have bullying at our school," was the response of the headmistress, peering at me over thick-rimmed spectacles.

"Every school has bullying," I snapped at her, "Only some schools fail to deal with it."

"If there has been bullying, Mrs Cunningham, of course we will look into it and the culprits, if found, will be punished," said the headmaster, tapping some papers on his desk. "Now about Louise's work, she is behind on every subject, failing on physics and often makes excuses for not handing in homework. This behaviour will not be tolerated at our school."

He sat back smugly in his chair, elbows on the arms and forming his long skinny fingers into a pyramid.

The headmistress sat there and yes, she was gloating. The head of year appeared to be studying her hands and Mrs Allan just looked miserable and uncomfortable.

"Maybe that's because she is being bullied," I said, determined not to be out flanked.

"I said we would deal with that, if it is in fact taking place."

"And I will deal with her low grade in physics and late homework, if it is in fact taking place." I interjected.

"Do you doubt me Msssss Cunningham?" Yes, he was hissing at me.

"Do you doubt my daughter?" I replied.

The meeting went from bad to worse, I was patronised and treated with disdain and I was too tired and emotional to deal with it adequately.

I drove away from the school, having hammered hell out of the starter motor of my car, much to the amusement of the 6th form rugby team, feeling angry and disappointed with my own inadequacy. I'd mentioned Lou's hair and the headmaster simply asked his colleagues if they had noticed anything, had they 'witnessed anyone pulling Louise's hair?', completely, and I believe deliberately, misconstruing what I had said.

Mrs Allan looked as if she wanted to say something but thought better of it and closed her mouth. I wished she had spoken, as I am sure it would have been in Lou's defence, but understood the difficulty of her position and accepted her silence.

Louise and I later discussed the one alternative – changing schools – but she, ever ambitious, was reluctant.
"It's a good school mum, I'll stick with it."

She did stick with it, for another two years, desperately unhappy and her hair pulling intensified. She had seen a mental health nurse and a psychologist at Keele but nothing made any difference and the worse thing was she changed.
I can only say that for a few months my Louise vanished and in her place was a moody, bad tempered, sullen, airhead. Everything was a performance. She floated around, calling David and I *dahling* and *de'ah* and referring to me as *mother dahling* something that really wound me up. She scoffed at things we said and insulted our intelligence, especially David's, getting short thrift from me.
I knew this wasn't just puberty, Lou had adopted an, 'if you can't beat them, join them' policy and it was unbearable.
Things came to crisis point one day when I was attempting to talk to her about her behaviour and she made to leave the room. I grabbed hold of her jumper and she ripped it out of my hand throwing me a challenging look before stomping out of the room.
I dashed after her, grabbed her and pinned her against the front door,

"You want to take me on madam, you want to break me?" I growled at her. "Your father tried that, hell, life has tried that and they both failed. You don't like the rules of this family, then pack a bag and go stay with the snooty friends you seem so impressed with and don't think of coming back until you are MY daughter again!"

I left her there and calmly walked back into the lounge where David was sitting white as a sheet. He had constantly been shocked by his sister's behaviour but now I believe he was shocked at mine.

It was loss of control on my part but she had pushed me to the limits. For weeks I had been allowing her some latitude but things were showing no sign of improving.

I winked at David and sat down noticing a look of relief on his face.

Lou appeared in the doorway,

"I'm so sorry mum," she wept, "I just don't know who I am any more. I try so hard to fit in but they just won't let me, then last week I was accused of trying to steal money and I've been so worried you'd find out."

"Tell me," I demanded, now alarmed at her obvious distress.

"After swimming, I wait for the others to go before I fix my hair, I don't want people seeing me take it down 'cos all my bald patches would show. You know I have that little tin with all my hair slides in"?

I nodded, I knew the tin well and often *topped* it up when I found the black slides she felt she needed to mask the bald patches.

"I was running late 'cos they were chatting and giggling and I thought they would never leave, so I was in a rush and I knocked the tin flying and the slides, they just flew everywhere and my hair was loose and I was just panicking, searching through all the bags on the floor, I needed them all mum, you know I needed them all."

"Calm down," I said nodding, pulling her next to me on the sofa and wiping her tears.

"Someone came in and saw me going through the bags, she said 'eeeeoooow look at the state of your hair' and walked out and the next thing I know I have to go to the headmaster's office and he accuses me of stealing. I had to apologise to everyone who had left a sports bag in there and say sorry for *trying* to steal from them, 'cos they hadn't found anything missing, but I hadn't done anything wrong."

She dissolved into more hysterical tears and I held her until she stopped crying.

I was beside myself with fury and in pain for my daughter. The school had played judge and jury and Lou had been punished in the cruellest way without them saying a word to me.

Taking her by the shoulders I made her look at me,

"That's it," I said, "We can't win this one, this school is simply NOT good enough for *you*, we'll find somewhere else but we won't go quietly, I promise you that, we are NOT going quietly"

Louise didn't return to that school but I did. The very next day I accosted the headmaster, outside his office. For once my timing was to perfection. Not only was it the last day of term, it was also open day and proud parents were passing by with their equally proud children.

For once I was 'power dressed' in Kate's/my cream trouser suit, a borrowed designer bag over my shoulder, looking every bit as wealthy as the parents passing by – hoping they wouldn't see me take the hammer to my car later.

He took my elbow and tried to steer me into his office but I pulled my arm away enjoying his embarrassment as he smiled at a passing family. In my best, most educated voice, I said …

"How dare you act as judge and jury over my child and punish her so cruelly for something you *thought* she was doing," I said, a little louder than necessary, glorifying in the interest taken by the visitors.

"I am removing her from this wretched school. I am removing her from a school that punishes the bullied and protects the bullies … oh forgive me you don't have bullying at YOUR school do you? Well, I'm sorry to say you *do* have it and it's running riot because you don't deal with it in fact you lead by example."

My heart pounding but determined to go on I turned to the small crowd of interested spectators that had formed nearby.

"Please step into my office Ms Cunningham, I'm sure it would be better to discuss this in private," said the now less confident, indeed panicking headmaster.

"No way," I laughed, "These people, who are probably going to pay massive fees for the privilege of sending their children to this school, have a perfect right to know a few things that are not in your glossy brochure."

Turning to the ever-growing audience and giving my best performance …

"My daughter, for three years, has been the victim of constant bullying, so much so she now self-harms, she pulls out, by the roots, her beautiful black hair. The school, not only denying that there is bullying, proceeded to intimidate me and then accused my daughter of *trying* to steal and without informing me, humiliated her in front of her peers."

I took from my bag a form the school had completed and approached the engrossed audience, which now included Mrs Allan and other teachers,

"This is a form the school had to complete before my daughter could receive any treatment for her condition. Let me read part of it to you. It asks: **'Please give, in the box below, any helpful information you may have on the above named child. If necessary, please use a second sheet of paper.'** The school's response to this: **'Failing at physics, some hair pulling."** I paused, reached into my bag and took out photographs of the top and back of Lou's head, her face not in view. They showed long dark silky hair but there was none at all on the top of her head. With tears in my eyes, I walked toward my now captivated audience and held the photographs out for them to see.

"*Some hair pulling*," I repeated, then, stepping over to the school notice board, which proudly displayed many of the school's success stories, I added the photographs of my child and walked away, my head held high.

I doubt my little one-woman performance made any difference. I did later hear that the headmaster had ripped the pictures from the notice board and thrown them in a nearby waste paper basket. When he was gone, a teacher picked them out and pinned them back on the board. I had touched one person's heart, maybe more. I also later heard that Mrs. Allan had resigned her position that same day.

Your children may break your heart but they also bring such joy and have the ability to make you laugh with the things they say and do with such innocence.

I recalled an elderly couple asking David what his young sister's name was,

"Louise" he said smiling proudly, "But mummy calls her 'Louise shut up.'" Then there was the time he took part in the school sports day and came running over to me after his race and announced, hugely pleased with himself,

"I came 4th! I came 4th! There had only been 4 in the race but David had just run, not bothering to look behind him. Good idea I thought.

Then there was the time I wanted to curl up and die. Earlier on in the day Lou and I had been sitting sorting out the ironing.

"These knickers of yours have to be washed again," she said frowning, looking at some of the underwear I kept purely for when I was menstruating. Knowing it would mean nothing to her, I replied,

"No those stains won't come out but I only wear them when I'm having my period."

Later on we were digging through clothing on sale in a local shop.

"How about this little dress?" I asked her, holding up a pretty flowered frock.

"No, I don't like it," she said shaking her head, "It's got a period on it!"

I recalled an occasion when I had to take her to hospital – she had an earring trapped in her nose.

She was only six and looked so tiny and vulnerable lying on a huge trolley, arms casually folded across her chest and legs crossed at the ankles, wearing her pink fluffy dressing gown and matching pink fluffy bunny rabbit slippers.

But when she raised her arms, signalled 'step back' and sat up, she sent everyone running for cover,

"Ah, ah, ah, ah, AHHHHH TISHOOOOO!!!!!!!!! …… OK get on with it," she casually commanded lying back down and folding her arms back across her chest.

With these happier memories euphoria returned and I drove back onto the motorway and headed south.

ESSEX HERE I COME
Growing old disgracefully?

Kate had arrived early. She had opened the windows and placed a beautiful vase of flowers on the windowsill of the bed-sit that was to be my new home. Outside David and Tony were struggling to get my bed around a corner and up two flights of stairs.

Kate and I hugged. We couldn't believe that I had finally made it home. We stood arms around each other surveying the small Essex County Council bed-sit, wondering how on earth I was going to cope.
"It's only until I can find somewhere more permanent," I assured her but didn't truly feel that confident. Prices in Essex were horrendous and although I was going to be earning a tad more than at Keele it was going to be a real struggle and I was reluctant to rent privately having been made homeless once.
So I was moving into a cheap, unexciting bed-sit, one of the few ECC rented out to employees moving into the area.
Nevertheless, I was really content. For the fist time in years I had only myself to think about.

There were four bed-sits on my floor but the others were empty so it was like having a large flat and outside there was a large garden with flowers and shrubs and trees and the beauty of it was, I didn't have to look after it … bliss. There was a small kitchen, a large lounge and dining room a bathroom and a separate shower and two toilets. My room had a large bay window and the first thing I did was put my own curtains up which immediately changed the dull, dreary atmosphere and when the sun shone through it was heaven. It was sparsely furnished but I added a few things of my own – my television and stereo, my computer, my own bed, lamps and lampshades and side tables on which I placed photographs and a few of my most precious ornaments. At night I lit candles which gave the room a warm, cosy ambience.

It was great getting home from work knowing I didn't have hours of cooking and cleaning ahead of me before bedtime. I only had to care for my own room, the rest of the floor was cleaned once a week by the ECC and it was so cheap, only my rent, no other bills.

For the first time in years I had money left in my account at the end of the month and I was able to indulge in that rare and wonderful thing, 'buying new clothes and shoes' and even dared to have a social life.

I loved my job and the fantastic caring people I worked with. It seemed everything I had worked so hard for at university, and even in previous jobs, had come together.

It was hard and it was stressful and the children I worked with were capable of breaking your heart. If I didn't already know it I soon discovered ... there are very few truly 'bad' children but there are far too many truly bad parents. In this day and age of computers and televisions, videos and DVD players and of course, pubs open all hours, children are often left to their own resources, being told to go and play and leave mum and dad in peace.

I recalled children of neighbours of mine in Madeley, banging on the door one night begging to be let in, only to be told by their parents to 'clear off and play' – children the same age as my own, who, unlike my neighbour's children, had been tucked up in their beds for almost two hours and were fast asleep.

As in so many stressful professions, we worked hard and we played hard – my social circle a crazy mixture of education welfare officers, mental health workers, probation officers, social workers, police officers, victim workers and many other administration staff, project workers and volunteers who came together under the umbrella of the Youth Offending Service. We partied hard but were forever vigilant; never overstepping the mark, aware that the young people we worked with could be monitoring and would maybe emulate our behaviour.

I also joined a few dating sites and was more than chuffed to discover that at 55 I could still attract men.

So I pubbed and clubbed and dated. Sometimes I wore short skirts – but never so short my daughter would disapprove and sometimes I wore low-necked tops – but never so low my son would disapprove. It wasn't so much 'growing old disgracefully' as 'living life to the full.'

Eventually I moved into a brand new, tiny, two bed roomed housing association flat, my clumsy second hand furniture looking very out of place, but I couldn't have cared less for I felt safe and secure, possibly for the first time in my life, and it is still my home to this day.

Money is still tight, especially as every vacation Lou returns home from Durham University to her mum. She applied to our local NHS Trust for expensive but proven treatment for her trichotillomania but was turned down ... their reason being and I quote

" ... *The Panel carefully considered all the information available to them but their decision was not to approve funding. It was felt that there was insufficient evidence to support that your patient had stopped hair pulling to the extent that they would benefit from any hair replacement treatment.*"

In other words, she had to *stop* pulling out her hair *before* they would agree to pay for treatment to *help her stop* pulling out her hair ... where, I ask, is the sense in that?!

David is happy and settled in the Midlands with his little family. Having struggled all his life academically, he studied and passed his electricians exams and can now proudly display the BSI (British Standards Institution) Kite mark logo.
He has battled with his drink problem and has stopped drinking alcohol altogether. He accepts he is an alcoholic, something his father never did, and for the sake of his partner and family, has fought to stop drinking and has finally succeeded.

I am so very, very proud of both my children, of their strength and resilience. Although we are far apart there is an invisible thread that binds us forever together and wraps us in warmth, mutual respect and love.

What has happened to me you may ask? Well, I would love to say that life finally became easier but in fact the menopause hit me hard and I have battled with bouts of depression. I have also found that, as you get older, you are more likely to be bullied at work and this has now happened to me twice. The second time I decided to fight back and, as I write, I am going through a long and drawn out dispute with the Essex County Council. It has been lonely and hard and friends and family have often wished I would give up but I just cannot, not this time. My boss made me so ill and I have suffered financially and emotionally. I wouldn't recommend anyone to take on such a large corporation alone. I have been lucky – my younger sister, Jane, has been with me every step of the way – without her I could not have continued. I will let you know, in my next book, how things worked out!!

In 1994 darling Pete, Kate's boyfriend, was killed in a dreadful road accident. He was only 28 and once again Kate and I were drawn together in grief. Sadly, in recent years, she and I have become estranged. We had been through so much together, so much sadness and so many struggles, that I think she needed to move on. I miss her every day but thank God for the friendship we shared. I will always be grateful for the love and support she gave me, so very many times and for so many years.

If you have bought my book and have read and enjoyed my story, maybe finding it funny, sad, helpful or thought provoking, then I will have truly achieved something very important to me. At the very least it will serve as a legacy to my children. It is a story of one woman's struggle against depression, poverty and adversity and it shows that, if you have the strength and the determination, you can rise above it all.

One night, if you are driving past a pub somewhere in Essex, you may hear a voice singing a well-known Frank Sinatra song. Although his and my life couldn't have been more different, like many of us I can share with him the sentiments of this song, and so you'll hear me singing, loudly and enthusiastically "*I faced it all and I stood tall and did it MY WAY*" ... and I will really, truly mean it!!

THE END